Field Guide to the Neurologic Examination

Field Guide *to* the Neurologic Examination

STEVEN L. LEWIS, M.D.

Associate Professor of Neurological Sciences
Head, Section of General Neurology
Neurology Residency Program Director
Department of Neurological Sciences
Rush Medical College of Rush University
Rush University Medical Center
Chicago, Illinois

LIPPINCOTT WILLIAMS & WILKINS
A **Wolters Kluwer** Company
Philadelphia · Baltimore · New York · London
Buenos Aires · Hong Kong · Sydney · Tokyo

Acquisitions Editor: Danette Somers
Developmental Editor: Tanya Lazar
Project Manager: Nicole Walz
Production Editor: Erica Broennle Nelson, Silverchair Science + Communications
Senior Manufacturing Manager: Benjamin Rivera
Cover Designer: Larry Didona
Compositor: Silverchair Science + Communications
Printer: R.R. Donnelley, Crawfordsville

© 2005 by LIPPINCOTT WILLIAMS & WILKINS
530 Walnut Street
Philadelphia, PA 19106 USA
LWW.com

Library of Congress Cataloging-in-Publication Data

Lewis, Steven L.
    Field guide to the neurologic examination / Steven L. Lewis.
      p ; cm. – (Field guide series)
    Includes bibliographical references and index.
    ISBN 0-7817-4186-6
      1. Neurologic examination. I. Title. II. Field guide (Philadelphia, Pa.)
    [DNLM: 1. Neurologic Examination—methods. WL 141 L676f 2004]
    RC348.L496 2004
    616.8'0475–dc22

                                                    2004011492

Care has been taken to confirm the accuracy of the information presented and to describe generally accepted practices. However, the authors, editors, and publisher are not responsible for errors or omissions or for any consequences from application of the information in this book and make no warranty, expressed or implied, with respect to the currency, completeness, or accuracy of the contents of the publication. Application of this information in a particular situation remains the professional responsibility of the practitioner.

The authors, editors, and publisher have exerted every effort to ensure that drug selection and dosage set forth in this text are in accordance with current recommendations and practice at the time of publication. However, in view of ongoing research, changes in government regulations, and the constant flow of information relating to drug therapy and drug reactions, the reader is urged to check the package insert for each drug for any change in indications and dosage and for added warnings and precautions. This is particularly important when the recommended agent is a new or infrequently employed drug.

Some drugs and medical devices presented in this publication have Food and Drug Administration (FDA) clearance for limited use in restricted research settings. It is the responsibility of health care providers to ascertain the FDA status of each drug or device planned for use in their clinical practice.

10 9 8 7 6 5 4 3 2 1

To my sons,
David, Michael, Adam, and Elliot

CONTENTS

PREFACE

The neurologic examination isn't an academic exercise. It's done to help figure out what's wrong with your patient.

This book explains how to perform the neurologic examination. But learning how to do the examination is of little value without understanding the purpose of the different components of the examination, knowing when these examination elements should be performed, recognizing what to look for, and understanding what the findings mean. This book attempts to teach the hows, whys, whens, and whats of the neurologic examination.

Elements of the neurologic examination that are of limited usefulness or relevance to modern neurologic diagnosis, or are too noxious with little benefit to be gained, are generally omitted from this text or are briefly described with a caveat of their limited role. For example, other than the Babinski sign, you won't find a description of multiple obscure ways, with equally obscure eponyms, to look for upper motor neuron signs in the feet. These additional signs are rarely useful or necessary. In the Cranial Nerve Examination section, you won't find a description of corneal reflex testing, because this noxious test is rarely indicated in an awake patient (corneal reflex testing is, however, described in a later chapter, Examination of the Comatose Patient).

This book is divided into three sections. The first section, Neurologic Diagnosis: General Considerations, is a general overview of the role of the neurologic history and examination in the diagnosis of patients with neurologic symptoms. The second section, Neurologic Examination, gives the nuts and bolts of why, when, and how to perform the different elements of the neurologic examination and how to interpret the results. The chapters in the third section, Neurologic Examination in Common Clinical Scenarios, discuss how to tailor the history and examination in different common clinical scenarios, depending on a patient's presenting symptoms. Examination elements that are specific to certain symptom complexes are described in these chapters.

My hope is that most readers will attempt to review the text in its entirety. On the other hand, this text is also meant to be used as a pocket reference, and readers should find this book helpful for looking up specific examination elements and basic information when needed in various clinical scenarios.

S.L.L.

ACKNOWLEDGMENTS

I'd like to thank Tanya Lazar, my editor at Lippincott Williams & Wilkins, for her expert guidance throughout the writing and production of this book, and Jennifer Smith for her talent and skill in turning my crude sketches and photographs into clear and instructive illustrations. I'd also like to thank the neurology residents at Rush University Medical Center for making teaching bedside clinical neurology so much fun, and my colleagues in the Department of Neurological Sciences, especially Jordan Topel, M.D., for being a clinical role model, and my chairman, Jacob H. Fox, M.D., for his support of neurologic education and general clinical neurology. Thanks also to Gail Valadez and Margaret Yesko, R.N., my administrative assistant and nurse, for making all my jobs so much easier and for being the model and photographer for the pictures on muscle strength and reflex testing from which the illustrations were drawn. Jack Cohen, M.D., director of the ophthalmology residency program at Rush, provided all of the fundus photographs for this text, for which I am very grateful.

Thank you to my mother for her encouragement throughout the years and for the personal sacrifices she made on my behalf. Finally, special thanks to my wife, Julie, for all of her support and for her patience and understanding for all the time spent away from my responsibilities at home while I wrote this book.

S.L.L.

Neurologic Diagnosis: General Considerations

Chapter 1

ROLE OF THE NEUROLOGIC HISTORY AND EXAMINATION IN NEUROLOGIC DIAGNOSIS

PURPOSE OF THE NEUROLOGIC HISTORY AND EXAMINATION

The purpose of the neurologic history and examination is to look for clues to the cause of a patient's neurologic symptoms. In neurologic diagnosis, this means that the history and examination are used to try to determine the localization of the disease process (i.e., where in the nervous system is the problem?), as well as the mechanism of the disease process (i.e., how is that problem occurring?), paving the way for the most appropriate diagnostic studies, if needed.

WHEN TO PERFORM THE NEUROLOGIC HISTORY AND EXAMINATION

A thorough neurologic history, followed by a neurologic examination, should be performed on all patients who present with symptoms suggestive of nervous system dysfunction.

NEUROANATOMY OF THE NEUROLOGIC HISTORY AND EXAMINATION

Neurologic disease can occur due to dysfunction anywhere in the peripheral or the central nervous system (see Chapter 2, Localization of Neurologic Disease).

EQUIPMENT NEEDED TO PERFORM THE NEUROLOGIC HISTORY AND EXAMINATION

Although not all items are necessary for every examination, the following are all of the items that you routinely need, so you really should make sure you have them:

- Ophthalmoscope
- Penlight (or the light of an otoscope)
- Pocket-sized visual acuity card
- A tongue depressor
- 512-Hz tuning fork
- 128-Hz tuning fork
- Reflex hammer

More information about these items and the clinical scenarios in which they are required can be found in Section 2, Neurologic Examination.

HOW TO PERFORM THE NEUROLOGIC HISTORY AND EXAMINATION

A neurologic history should always be performed first, followed by the neurologic examination. Any other order is fraught with hazard in the quest for the correct clinical diagnosis and is much less efficient.

During the history, the examiner should be attempting to hone the diagnostic considerations, so that by the time the history is complete, the most likely and unlikely localizations and mechanisms of the patient's problem should be evident. A thorough neurologic examination is then performed with the intent of searching for clues to support or refute the diagnostic hypotheses developed from the history.

The specific elements of the thorough neurologic examination may vary, however, depending on the patient's presenting symptoms. Knowing what you are looking for during the examination, based on the findings from the history, allows you to include otherwise optional examination elements that may be useful to answer the specific diagnostic questions that are being entertained. Throughout this book, the usefulness, or lack thereof, of examination elements in different clinical scenarios is stressed. There are certain parts of the neurologic examination, however, that should be performed on all new patients who present with a neurologic complaint (see Chapter 40, Performing a Complete Neurologic Examination) or as part of a routine complete general medical examination in patients who have no neurologic complaints (see Chapter 53, Examination of the Patient without Neurologic Symptoms: The Screening Neurologic Examination).

NORMAL FINDINGS

Patients without neurologic disease usually have normal neurologic examinations; however, many patients with neurologic disease, particularly those patients with transient symptoms, also have normal neurologic examinations. This underscores the added importance of the neurologic history in these patients.

It is also not uncommon for patients who do not have neurologic symptoms or underlying neurologic disease to have subtle findings that may be clinically insignificant. Although it takes a fair amount of clinical experience to be comfortable in knowing when to discard these incidental findings, the author's hope is that readers of this book will be a step closer to this important aspect of neurologic diagnosis.

Throughout this book, each examination element is summarized with a description of its normal finding.

ABNORMAL FINDINGS

Many patients with neurologic disease, particularly those with persistent (not transient) symptoms, have abnormal neurologic examinations that provide clues to the diagnosis.

Throughout this book, individual components of the examination are described with a description of the significant abnormal findings for each, as well as a discussion of the most likely interpretations of these findings.

ADDITIONAL POINTS

- Always take the neurologic history before performing the neurologic examination.
- While you proceed with the neurologic history and neurologic examination, always try to think about the localization of neurologic dysfunction (see Chapter 2, Localization of Neurologic Disease) before thinking about the mechanism of that dysfunction (see Chapter 3, Mechanisms of Neurologic Disease).

LOCALIZATION OF NEUROLOGIC DISEASE

PURPOSE OF NEUROLOGIC LOCALIZATION

The purpose of neurologic localization—an essential component of neurologic diagnosis—is to determine where in the nervous system the patient's dysfunction is occurring, paving the way for the second key element of neurologic diagnosis, the determination of the mechanism of that dysfunction (see Chapter 3, Mechanisms of Neurologic Disease).

WHEN TO PERFORM NEUROLOGIC LOCALIZATION

Neurologic localization needs to be performed in every patient who presents with a symptom that is potentially due to nervous system dysfunction. Localization is often not hard, especially if you initially think in terms of the gross neuroanatomic areas described in this chapter and don't try to overcomplicate things. Neurologic localization is a thought process that should occur during and after every neurologic history and during and after every neurologic examination.

NEUROANATOMY OF NEUROLOGIC LOCALIZATION

Neurologic disease can occur due to dysfunction anywhere within the central or peripheral nervous system. The nervous system can be divided into eight major areas as listed in Box 2–1, and these are the regions to which you should initially try to localize neurologic disease. Although narrower localization is clearly optimal (i.e., *where* in the brain or spinal cord is the problem?), you've made a lot of headway if you can decide in which of these eight major areas your patient's problem most likely resides.

The diagnostic importance of the ability to localize your patient's neurologic dysfunction to one of these gross neuroanatomic regions should not be underestimated. Table 2–1 summarizes some of the diagnostically relevant functions of these eight regions of the nervous system; in Table 2–1, the brain (cerebral hemispheres) is subdivided into the cerebral hemispheric cortex and the deep cerebral hemisphere.

EQUIPMENT NEEDED TO LOCALIZE NEUROLOGIC DISEASE

None (other than the equipment used for the neurologic examination—localization is a thought process).

HOW TO LOCALIZE NEUROLOGIC DISEASE

Localization is based on the symptoms obtained from the history and the signs found during the neurologic examination. The process of localization consists of deciding which area of nervous system dysfunction best explains these symptoms and signs based on knowledge of the function of these regions. Table 2–2 summarizes some symptoms and signs that are helpful in localizing neurologic disease to the general regions of the nervous system.

BOX 2–1	**General Locations of Nervous System Disease**

Central Nervous System
Brain (cerebral hemispheres)[a]
Brainstem
Cerebellum
Spinal cord

Peripheral Nervous System
Nerve root
Peripheral nerve[b] (including most cranial nerves[c])
Neuromuscular junction
Muscle

[a]Although the brainstem and cerebellum are technically part of the brain, most clinicians think of "the brain" as the cerebral hemispheres without the brainstem and cerebellum.
[b]The brachial plexus and the lumbar plexus would be included within the "peripheral nerve" localization.
[c]Most of the cranial nerves are peripheral nerves, except for cranial nerves I and II, which are actually extensions of the central nervous system.

These principles and the use of signs and symptoms to further narrow the regions of localization are described in greater detail throughout this book.

NORMAL FINDINGS

Patients without neurologic disease have nothing to localize.

ABNORMAL FINDINGS

The abnormal finding on neurologic localization is the region of localization itself. During the diagnostic process, the localization can be reported broadly (e.g., left hemisphere or spinal cord) or narrowly (e.g., left temporal lobe or cervical spinal cord) as you feel is most appropriate given the clues from the history and examination and the outcome of investigations.

TABLE 2–1 Simplified Listing of Some Diagnostically Relevant Functions of the Major Regions of the Nervous System

Region	Some Major Functions of the Region
Brain (hemispheric cortex)	Thought, language, memory, visual perception of contralateral space, contralateral motor and sensory function
Brain (deep cerebral hemisphere)	Contralateral motor and sensory function
Brainstem	Eye movements, motor and sensory function of face and body, alertness, sensation of nausea, coordination of extremities, balance
Cerebellum	Coordination of extremities, balance
Spinal cord	Motor and sensory function of the body and extremities, bowel and bladder control
Nerve root	Motor and sensory function in territory of nerve root
Peripheral nerve (or cranial nerve)	Motor and sensory function in territory of nerve or cranial nerve
Neuromuscular junction	Motor function of extremities, eye movements, swallowing, breathing
Muscle	Motor function

TABLE 2-2 Characteristic Symptoms and Signs of Neurologic Disease at Different Major Locations

General Location	Characteristic Symptoms and Signs Suggestive of Localization to This Region[a]
Brain (hemispheric cortex)	Cognitive dysfunction
	Speech and language dysfunction
	Hemiparesis
	Hemisensory loss
	Visual field deficits
	Headache
	Upper motor neuron signs
Brain (deep hemisphere)	Hemiparesis
	Hemisensory loss
	Headache
	Upper motor neuron signs
Brainstem	Diplopia, dysarthria, nausea, vomiting, vertigo
	Alterations in level of consciousness
	Ataxia of gait or extremities
	Unilateral or bilateral weakness or sensory loss
	Crossed hemiparesis (e.g., weakness on one side of the face and the opposite side of the body)
	Crossed hemisensory loss (numbness on one side of the face and the opposite side of the body)
	Upper motor neuron signs
Cerebellum	Ataxia of gait or extremities
	Dysarthria, nausea, vomiting, vertigo
	Headache
Spinal cord	Bilateral weakness and sensory loss
	Bowel and bladder dysfunction
	Brown-Séquard syndrome (see Chapter 51, Examination of the Patient with a Suspected Spinal Cord Problem)
	Upper motor neuron signs
Nerve root	Radiating pain corresponding to a nerve root distribution
	Numbness or weakness in a nerve root distribution
	Diminished reflex (lower motor neuron signs) in territory of nerve root
Peripheral nerve	Distal paresthesias, sensory loss, or weakness
	Diminished distal reflexes (distal lower motor neuron signs)
Neuromuscular junction	Waxing and waning weakness, dysarthria, dysphagia, ptosis, diplopia
Muscle	Weakness (especially proximal)

[a]Not all lesions in these locations produce these symptoms and signs; however, the finding of these symptoms and signs would be consistent with this localization.

Some areas of localization have their own neurologic terminology to describe them. These useful terms, which are listed and defined in Table 2–3, are helpful in categorizing sites of neurologic dysfunction. Because these terms are generic and only imply broad localization, a causative process is not implied; the only implication is that there is pathology of some sort (hence the suffix -*opathy*) involving that structure.

TABLE 2-3 Common Terms Used to Describe Localizations of Neurologic Dysfunction

Term	Meaning	Origin of Prefix	Comments
Encephalopathy	Disease of brain	*Encephalo*: brain	Refers to diffuse, not focal, brain dysfunction
Myelopathy	Disease of spinal cord	*Myelo*: spinal cord	Refers to any cause of spinal cord dysfunction
Radiculopathy	Disease of nerve root	*Radiculo*: root	Refers to any cause of nerve root dysfunction
Neuropathy	Disease of nerve	*Neuro*: nerve	Refers to any cause of nerve dysfunction
Myopathy	Disease of muscle	*Myo*: muscle	Refers to any cause of muscle dysfunction

ADDITIONAL POINTS

- Localization is the key to neurologic diagnosis; it's why we're taught neuroanatomy in medical school.
- The neuroanatomy that you need to know to localize neurologic disease is not really that much (less than what you were taught in medical school)! The important basic pathways (and shortcuts) that you need to know for neurologic localization and for understanding the role of each component of the examination are described throughout this book.

Chapter 3

MECHANISMS OF NEUROLOGIC DISEASE

PURPOSE

The purpose of determining the mechanism of neurologic disease is to come closer to a patient's diagnosis by determining the cause of the patient's neurologic dysfunction. By determining how the dysfunction is occurring, the second part of the neurologic diagnostic process is complete (after localization; see Chapter 2, Localization of Neurologic Disease), giving a more complete picture of the neurologic diagnosis.

WHEN TO DETERMINE THE MECHANISM OF NEUROLOGIC DISEASE

An attempt to determine the mechanism of neurologic disease needs to be made in every patient who presents with a symptom due to nervous system dysfunction. Determination of mechanism is a thought process that should occur during and after every neurologic history, and during and after every neurologic examination.

NEUROANATOMY OF DISEASE MECHANISM

Determination of mechanism is based less directly on neuroanatomy than is localization (see Chapter 2, Localization of Neurologic Disease). Mechanism is intertwined in localization (and, therefore, neuroanatomy), however, because your choice of mechanisms is limited to those processes that are likely to affect that region of the nervous system.

EQUIPMENT NEEDED TO DETERMINE THE MECHANISM OF NEUROLOGIC DISEASE

None (other than the equipment used for the neurologic examination—the determination of mechanism is a thought process).

HOW TO DETERMINE THE MECHANISM OF NEUROLOGIC DISEASE

In neurologic diagnosis, it is most helpful to think in terms of general mechanisms of neurologic dysfunction and to try to decide which of these mechanisms is likely to be causative before proceeding with further diagnostic studies. Table 3–1 lists the major categories of neurologic disease mechanism. These mechanisms are generic and broad; for example, the compressive mechanism would include diverse disease processes, such as a tumor compressing or infiltrating brain tissue, a thoracic disc compressing the spinal cord, or a subdural hematoma causing mass effect on the brain. The same pathologic process can even produce clinical symptoms through several different mechanisms; for example, an intracerebral aneurysm may produce disease when it bleeds or when it compresses important structures (e.g., a posterior communicating artery aneurysm causing a compressive oculomotor nerve palsy).

TABLE 3–1 General Mechanisms of Neurologic Disease[a]

Mechanism	Comments
Compressive	Includes any processes that produce dysfunction by compression of nervous system structures [e.g., tumors (benign or malignant), intervertebral discs compressing nerve roots or spinal cord, aneurysm compressing a cranial nerve]
Degenerative	Includes any process that causes progressive dysfunction due to nervous system degeneration; this mechanism is especially causative in many dementing illnesses (e.g., Alzheimer's disease and other degenerative dementias), many movement disorders (e.g., Parkinson's disease, Huntington's disease), and some neuromuscular diseases (e.g., amyotrophic lateral sclerosis)
Demyelinative	May involve central nervous system myelin (e.g., multiple sclerosis) or peripheral nervous system myelin (e.g., demyelinative peripheral neuropathies, such as Guillain-Barré syndrome); demyelinative disorders often have accompanying inflammation—think of *demyelinative* as a subset of *inflammatory* etiologies
Epileptic	Produces dysfunction by abnormal electrical activity of cerebral hemispheric cortex
Hemorrhagic	Produces dysfunction by bleeding into the brain or other tissues (e.g., intraparenchymal brain hemorrhage, intraventricular hemorrhage, subarachnoid hemorrhage)
Infectious	Dysfunction occurring due to a microorganism (e.g., bacterial, viral, parasitic) invading nervous system structures; probably best thought of as a subset of inflammatory etiologies
Inflammatory	Dysfunction occurring as a result of any inflammatory process involving the central or peripheral nervous system (e.g., autoimmune, granulomatous)
Ischemic	Dysfunction due to insufficient blood supply in the central nervous system (e.g., brain, brainstem, cerebellar, or spinal cord ischemia or infarction) or the peripheral nervous system (e.g., infarction of a peripheral nerve)
Migrainous	Mechanism of brain dysfunction that is thought to be due to spreading waves of depression of cortical activity; can lead to migrainous visual, motor, sensory, or aphasic symptoms, even in the absence of headache
Metabolic (including toxic)	Mechanism of diffuse brain or brainstem dysfunction due to effect of endogenous metabolic abnormalities (e.g., hyponatremia, hepatic or uremic dysfunction) or exogenous toxins (e.g., medications)
Traumatic	Central or peripheral nervous system dysfunction due to any kind of traumatic disruption of these structures

[a]In addition to the mechanisms in this list, some congenital processes may produce dysfunction due to the absence, malformation, or other developmental abnormality of nervous system structure or function since birth (whether on a microscopic or macroscopic level); this mechanism is most common with pediatric neurologic diagnoses.

The most important clues to the disease mechanism derive from the time course of symptom development discovered from the neurologic history. Neurologic symptoms can be transient—usually meaning lasting from seconds to hours—or persistent. Persistent symptoms can begin suddenly (and continue at the same severity or ultimately improve), progress gradually from onset, or wax and wane. Although the temporal pattern of symptom development is not specific for a single mechanism, these temporal patterns of symp-

TABLE 3–2   Historical Clues to Disease Mechanism Suggested by the Temporal Pattern of Symptom Development[a]

Temporal Course	Distribution	Most Likely Mechanisms
Transient (lasting seconds to hours)	Focal	Focal cerebral ischemia
		Migraine
		Focal seizure
	Diffuse	Global cerebral ischemia
		Generalized seizure
		Toxic/metabolic
Sudden onset (may have gradual improvement over variable period after onset)	Focal or diffuse	Ischemia (especially embolic)
		Hemorrhage
Gradually progressive (usually over hours, days, or longer; may also wax and wane)	Focal	Compressive
		Demyelinative
		Ischemic (especially thrombotic)
		Infectious
		Inflammatory
	Diffuse	Degenerative[b]
		Infectious
		Inflammatory
		Toxic/metabolic

[a]Many of the processes listed here would be expected to recur in a patient (e.g., seizures, migraine, demyelination in multiple sclerosis); this table refers to the time course of individual symptom development, not necessarily the overall course of a disease process.
[b]Most degenerative processes are progressive over months to years.

tom development can be quite helpful in including or excluding some of these mechanisms. Table 3–2 lists some of the mechanisms suggested by different temporal courses of neurologic symptoms, coupled with the additional information—obtained by history and examination—about whether the dysfunction is focal or diffuse.

NORMAL FINDINGS

Patients without neurologic disease have no mechanism of disease to determine.

ABNORMAL FINDINGS

The mechanism of disease that you uncover is the abnormal finding. During the diagnostic process, the mechanism can be reported broadly (e.g., ischemia) or narrowly (e.g., ischemia due to a high-grade carotid artery stenosis), as is most appropriate given the clues from the history and examination and the outcome of investigations.

The mechanism of disease is the adjective that goes in front of the localization. For example, a patient with a myelopathy (spinal cord dysfunction) as the localization of neurologic pathology can have a compressive myelopathy (e.g., from disc or tumor), an ischemic myelopathy (e.g., an anterior spinal artery infarct), or an inflammatory or demyelinative myelopathy (e.g., transverse myelitis). In the last example, sometimes a suffix is added to the region of localization to imply a mechanism. Specifically, the suffix -itis can be added when appropriate to invoke an inflammatory process as the cause of dysfunction at a particular localization [e.g., an inflammatory myelopathy is a *myelitis*, an inflammatory myopathy (muscle disease) can be reported as a *myositis*, and an inflammatory brain process can be called an *encephalitis*].

ADDITIONAL POINTS

- The determination of disease mechanism is highly dependent on the clues obtained from the history.
- Understanding the mechanism of dysfunction is the key to the treatment of disease or to the prevention of further disease. For example, the treatment of brain dysfunction due to compression is significantly different than the treatment of brain dysfunction due to ischemia. In addition, the prevention of further brain ischemia differs if the ischemia is due to cardiogenic embolism or carotid artery stenosis.
- Before attempting to determine the mechanism of dysfunction, make sure you have tried to localize that dysfunction. You can't determine the mechanism of dysfunction if you don't have some idea of where the problem is.

Neurologic Examination
Neurologic History

Chapter 4

TAKING A NEUROLOGIC HISTORY

PURPOSE

The purpose of the neurologic history—the most important component of neurologic evaluation—is to obtain information helpful in determining the localization and the mechanism of the patient's disease process.

WHEN TO PERFORM THE NEUROLOGIC HISTORY

A thorough neurologic history should be performed on all patients who present with symptoms suggestive of nervous system dysfunction. The history should always be taken before the examination is performed.

NEUROANATOMY OF THE NEUROLOGIC HISTORY

See Chapter 2, Localization of Neurologic Disease.

EQUIPMENT NEEDED TO PERFORM THE NEUROLOGIC HISTORY

None.

HOW TO PERFORM THE NEUROLOGIC HISTORY

Introduction

1. Greet the patient.
2. Sit down and make yourself—the examiner—comfortable. Don't be hurried or cut corners; reserve enough time for this important part of neurologic evaluation (obviously in the rare, truly emergent situation, you need to make yourself less comfortable and take a rapid, pointed, judicious history).
3. Take the history from the patient first, if possible, before talking to family members or other witnesses.

Chief Complaint

1. Don't assume that you know why the patient is seeing you or what the complaint or problem is.
2. After greeting the patient, discern the patient's chief complaint by asking the patient a general question, such as "What brings you here today?" Listen carefully to the patient's response.

History of Present Illness

1. Once you have an idea of what the main complaint is, take your time to define the specific details of the patient's history.

2. Ask the patient to start at the beginning and tell you the story. If the problem began yesterday morning, ask the patient to tell you the details, starting perhaps with the night before. If the history is of recurrent events dating back weeks, months, or years, try to get the specific details of each episode starting from the initial one.

3. After listening to the patient tell the history, ask specific, clarifying questions so you can better understand the patient's symptoms:

   • Elucidate the nature of the patient's symptoms by asking the patient to describe them. Symptoms such as weakness, numbness, and dizziness can mean different things to different patients at different times. When necessary, clarify the patient's symptom by asking something like, "What do you mean by . . . ?" Try not to put words into the patient's mouth; however, if you still have a difficult time understanding the nature of the patient's symptoms, you may have to give the patient multiple choices to define his or her symptoms.

   • Ask about the quality and intensity of symptoms. This is particularly appropriate for the complaint of pain, which may, for example, be sharp, dull, throbbing, or lancinating.

   • Ask about the timing and duration of the symptoms. Was the onset sudden or gradual? Did the symptoms resolve and, if so, how quickly? Have the symptoms been progressively worsening or improving, or waxing and waning?

   • What was the patient doing when the symptoms began or when the symptoms occur? Did the symptoms begin during rest or during exertion? If the symptoms are intermittent, do they occur more often in certain positions, such as while standing or lying down?

   • Ask the patient to point to the area of involvement, particularly when there is a sensory symptom or pain.

   • Are there any factors that make the symptoms better or worse?

4. Ask about the presence or absence of additional neurologic or systemic symptoms that may help you diagnostically in the given clinical scenario, as described in the chapters in Section 3, Neurologic Examination in Common Clinical Scenarios. Don't just mechanically ask historical details while you take the history, however. Remember that you're trying to figure out what's wrong with the patient by finding historical clues to the localization and the pathogenesis of the disease process. Think about what the information could be telling you about what might or might not be causing the patient's symptoms as you listen to the patient and formulate questions.

5. If appropriate, with the patient's permission, corroborate historical details or learn new historical details from family members or other witnesses to the problem. Although information volunteered from family members or friends accompanying the patient can be helpful, when you ask the patient a subjective question about the quality of a symptom that only the patient can really answer (e.g., "What do you mean by numbness?"), don't let anyone else answer for the patient. Of course, if the patient is unable to give any history (e.g., due to impairment of cognition or loss of consciousness), all of the history may need to be obtained from others.

The Rest of the Story

As in any medical evaluation, complete the history by obtaining the following:

- *Past medical history:* Ask the patient about any chronic illnesses, other previous illnesses, previous hospitalizations, and operations.
- *Medications:* Ask the patient about any medications he or she may be taking. Don't forget to ask about over-the-counter medications, herbal preparations, and, in women, oral contraceptives; many patients forget to include these when asked to list their medications.
- *Allergies:* Ask the patient about allergies to medications or other significant allergies. Also ask about any other previous adverse reactions to medications.
- *Social history:* Learn about the patient. What is the patient's occupation and educational background? Is the patient currently working, retired, or disabled? Ask about the home situation: Is the patient single, married, divorced, or widowed? How many children, if any, does the patient have? Has there been any recent stress? Don't just limit your social history to asking about tobacco, alcohol, and drug use—learning about the patient as a person is interesting, may give important diagnostic clues, may tell you information about cognitive baseline (when appropriate), and is important in assessing social support.
- *Family history:* Ask about any significant illnesses (neurologic or otherwise) in the patient's parents, grandparents, siblings, and children. Ask the patient specifically whether there is a family history of the particular illnesses that you feel are important to be aware of in the clinical scenario.
- *Review of systems:* As in any medical history, the initial evaluation of any patient should include an appropriate and extensive review of systems; this, of course, should not be limited to the neurologic system. Significant clues to the cause of a patient's problem may be found here, but do watch out for red herrings.

NORMAL FINDINGS

Patients without neurologic disease have no neurologic history to obtain.

ABNORMAL FINDINGS

See Chapter 2, Localization of Neurologic Disease, and Chapter 3, Mechanisms of Neurologic Disease, for discussions on using clues from the neurologic history to determine the localization and mechanism of neurologic disease.

ADDITIONAL POINTS

- Although this book devotes only one chapter specifically to the neurologic history, the neurologic history is the single most important component of neurologic evaluation. Without first taking an appropriate history, the examination is of extremely limited value and the interpretation (and selection of) diagnostic studies is fraught with peril.
- Sometimes you need to aggressively search for the appropriate witnesses to the patient's event to clarify the history. For example, if a patient presents because of an episode of loss of consciousness that occurred at a store, call the store to try to locate and speak to the individual who witnessed the problem. Think and act like a detective when searching for historical clues. Taking a few extra minutes to clarify the history from a firsthand witness can ultimately save time and prevent unnecessary investigations.

- When using an interpreter, ask the question to the patient and let the interpreter translate your question to the patient and directly translate the patient's response. The interpreter should avoid simply paraphrasing the patient or giving a subjective interpretation of what he or she thinks the patient's answer might mean medically. The interpreter is there only to translate the patient's language; your job is to translate the patient's history and examination into a diagnosis.

Chapter 5

APPROACH TO THE MENTAL STATUS EXAMINATION

PURPOSE

The purpose of the examination of mental status is to look for evidence of disorders that can affect the level of consciousness (alertness) or any aspect of cognitive function.

WHEN TO PERFORM THE MENTAL STATUS EXAMINATION

Mental status should be informally assessed in all patients simply by observing and listening to the patient while you are taking the history. Formal evaluation of mental status should be performed when there is a clinical suspicion or complaint of a cognitive problem, or when there appears to be a decrease in the patient's level of consciousness.

NEUROANATOMY OF THE MENTAL STATUS

Level of Consciousness

To be awake and alert requires intactness of at least one of the cerebral hemispheres, as well as the upper brainstem from the middle of the pons and above (see Chapter 42, Examination of the Comatose Patient).

Cognition

Cognition is a general term referring to mental abilities, such as memory, language, orientation, knowledge, and other aspects of intellectual functioning. Some cognitive abilities have well-recognized neuroanatomic localization, such as language to the dominant cerebral hemispheric cortex (see Chapter 6, Language Testing) or memory to the medial temporal lobes and thalami (see Chapter 7, Memory Testing); most other cognitive functions, however, although known to involve the cortex, are not clinically localizable to a specific neuroanatomic area.

EQUIPMENT NEEDED TO PERFORM THE MENTAL STATUS EXAMINATION

None (except paper and a pen or pencil).

HOW TO EXAMINE MENTAL STATUS

See Chapter 6, Language Testing; Chapter 7, Memory Testing; and Chapter 8, Testing Orientation, Concentration, Knowledge, and Constructional Ability for additional information.

NORMAL FINDINGS

Normally, patients should be awake and alert, fully oriented, have no impairment of language or memory, and have intellectual functioning compatible with their level of education and occupation.

ABNORMAL FINDINGS

Level of Consciousness

Changes in the level of consciousness from drowsiness to coma can occur due to dysfunction of both cerebral hemispheres, dysfunction of the upper brainstem (from the middle of the pons or above), or the combination of hemispheric and upper brainstem dysfunction (see Chapter 42, Examination of the Comatose Patient).

Cognition

- Changes in cognition can occur due to dysfunction anywhere within the cerebral hemispheres. Cognitive changes generally do not occur with lesions of the brainstem.
- Dysfunction of language (see Chapter 6, Language Testing) usually occurs due to a lesion within the dominant hemisphere.
- Disorders of memory (see Chapter 7, Memory Testing) tend to occur due to dysfunction of the medial temporal lobes or the thalami.
- Patients with the cognitive deficit of neglect of the left side of space, such as ignoring the left side of a figure when drawing (see Chapter 8, Testing Orientation, Concentration, Knowledge, and Constructional Ability), or ignoring the left side of their body, have dysfunction of their right (usually nondominant) hemisphere.
- Other cognitive problems, such as confusion and problems with orientation and knowledge (see Chapter 8, Testing Orientation, Concentration, Knowledge, and Constructional Ability), may not be localizable to a specific anatomic lesion and are likely due to multifocal or diffuse brain dysfunction.
- Impairment of processes such as judgment, mood, or the perception of reality (e.g., psychosis) can occur due to psychiatric disorders (in which the discrete neuroanatomic or physiologic lesion causing such symptoms is generally unknown), although similar symptoms can occur as a result of diffuse brain dysfunction associated with dementing illnesses or acute encephalopathies (delirium).

ADDITIONAL POINTS

- Changes in cognition can and usually do occur without necessarily affecting the level of consciousness. For example, patients with chronic dementia usually have normal alertness despite significant deterioration in cognitive functioning.
- Standardized batteries of mental status testing are used by many clinicians to screen patients for cognitive impairment, particularly in the setting of possible dementia. The most commonly used of these is the Folstein Mini-Mental State Examination, which uses a series of tasks to assess multiple areas of cognition. This test can give a somewhat quantitative score of global cognitive function, which can be followed serially to assess for worsening or improvement in the patient's symptoms. In the undiagnosed patient with a disorder of mental status, however, it is the assessment of the patient's ability to perform the specific individual components of

mental status testing (whether part of a standardized battery or not) that is of greatest diagnostic significance when attempting to localize and diagnose a potentially focal neurologic disease process.

- Cognitive testing should always be interpreted within the context of the patient's baseline level of intellectual functioning, as determined by the information obtained from the history (through the patient and family) about factors such as the patient's educational status and occupation.

Chapter 6

LANGUAGE TESTING

PURPOSE

The purpose of language testing is to look for evidence of dysfunction of the hemispheric cortical regions that are involved in the production or comprehension of spoken or written language.

WHEN TO TEST LANGUAGE

The ability of your patient to understand and produce spoken language should be evident by informal observation during the history and throughout your interaction with the patient. More formal evaluation of language function should be performed when there is a complaint of difficulty with language or speech, or when you suspect a disorder of language from your conversation with the patient during the history. In addition, language function should be tested in any patient with a right hemiparesis to look for evidence of localization of the neurologic process to the cortex.

NEUROANATOMY OF LANGUAGE

Language function resides in the left hemispheric cortex in essentially all right-handed patients and at least one-half of left-handed patients. The side of the brain where a patient's language is located is called the *dominant hemisphere*.

There are two main areas of the dominant hemisphere that are important for language function: Broca's area and Wernicke's area. Broca's area is located in the inferior frontal lobe, just anterior to the motor cortex, and is involved in the production of language. Wernicke's area is located in the posterior-superior temporal lobe, near the auditory cortex, and is involved in the comprehension of language.

EQUIPMENT NEEDED TO TEST LANGUAGE

None.

HOW TO EXAMINE LANGUAGE

1. Listen to the patient's spontaneous speech (this can be done while you are taking the history). Assess whether the speech is fluent and meaningful, if there are any errors in producing individual words, and if there are any unusual or nonexistent words. Also note if there is any problem with articulation (i.e., slurring) of speech.

If more formal language evaluation is necessary (see When to Test Language), proceed further:

2. Ask the patient to name one or a few commonly available objects, such as a pen, a watch, or a tie. Hold the object in front of the patient and ask, "What is this called?" After the patient has named the object, ask the patient to name one or two smaller parts of the object, such as the cap of the pen, the stem (or winder) or the wristband of the watch, or the knot of the tie. Having the patient name smaller parts of the objects is a more difficult task than simply naming only the object itself and may uncover aphasic errors that would not otherwise be evident.

3. Ask the patient to repeat a sentence after you have said it, such as "I am in the hospital" or any sentence of your choice. It is also helpful to ask the patient to repeat the phrase "no ifs, ands, or buts," because this kind of phrase is particularly difficult for aphasic patients to say.
4. Give the patient a sheet of paper and a pen or pencil and ask the patient to write any sentence of his or her choice.
5. Hand the patient a magazine or brochure (or other nontechnical material available nearby) and ask the patient to read a few sentences to you.

NORMAL FINDINGS

Normally, patients should be able to speak fluently, appropriately, and clearly, to comprehend spoken and written language well, and to name and repeat.

ABNORMAL FINDINGS

Two kinds of abnormalities may be found when assessing speech: aphasia or dysarthria. Patients who are aphasic have a problem with the production or comprehension of spoken or written language due to dysfunction of brain regions important for language. Patients who are dysarthric do not have language dysfunction, but they have speech that is slurred and inarticulate; this is due simply to a problem with control of the structures that move the mouth or tongue.

Aphasias

Broca's Aphasia (Also Called Motor or Expressive Aphasia)

- The speech of patients with Broca's aphasia is nonfluent, with obvious hesitancy and pauses between words and grammatic errors. The words that are produced, although hesitant and produced with difficulty, are generally correct, but there may be paraphasic errors. Paraphasic errors are words that are produced with inappropriate substitutions of parts of the words, such as saying "lencil" for "pencil."
- Patients with Broca's aphasia generally have intact ability to comprehend written and spoken language and to follow commands, but they do have difficulty repeating phrases.
- Patients with Broca's aphasia often say something like (although hesitantly and nonfluently) "I know what I want to say but I can't get the words out," and they usually appear frustrated because of their awareness of their difficulty communicating.
- Broca's aphasia occurs because of a lesion at or near Broca's area in the dominant frontal lobe. There is often an accompanying hemiparesis because of the proximity of Broca's area to the motor strip.

Wernicke's Aphasia (Also Called Sensory or Receptive Aphasia)

- The speech of patients with Wernicke's aphasia is fluent but makes little if any sense. Their speech is filled with nonsensical words and neologisms ("new words" that do not really exist in the patient's language), unusual combinations of words, and paraphasic errors.
- Patients with Wernicke's aphasia have poor comprehension but have little awareness of this; therefore, they produce strings of fluent, unusual sentences without the frustration seen in patients with Broca's aphasia. Like patients with Broca's aphasia, patients with Wernicke's aphasia also have difficulty with repetition.
- Wernicke's aphasia occurs because of a lesion at or near Wernicke's area in the dominant temporal lobe. Because of the distance of Wernicke's

area from the motor strip, patients with Wernicke's aphasia often do not have an associated hemiparesis. The only additional finding that may be found (although not always easily detected) in patients with Wernicke's aphasia is a right upper quadrant visual field deficit, due to the passage of these visual pathway fibers through the temporal lobe (see Chapter 13, Visual Field Examination).

Dysarthria

- Patients who are dysarthric have slurring of their speech but have no problem with language function. They can name, read, comprehend, and repeat but simply have poorly articulated speech that, depending on the severity of the dysarthria, can be difficult to understand.
- Dysarthria can occur due to dysfunction anywhere in the brain, brainstem, or cerebellum; therefore, the finding of dysarthria may not be helpful in specific neurologic localization. Dysarthria can also occur due to nonneurologic processes, such as any local cause of dysfunction of the mouth or tongue.
- Severe dysarthria particularly occurs in the setting of a *pseudobulbar palsy.* In addition to a marked "explosive" spastic dysarthria, patients with this syndrome usually have dysphagia and emotional lability. Pseudobulbar palsies occur due to bilateral lesions (e.g., due to multiple sclerosis or strokes) of the cerebral hemispheres, internal capsule, or upper brainstem affecting the corticobulbar tracts.

ADDITIONAL POINTS

- Because patients with Wernicke's aphasia often don't have other obvious findings on examination, and because the fluent speech disorder of Wernicke's aphasia is so unusual, patients with Wernicke's aphasia are often misdiagnosed as having a psychiatric disorder. Think about the possibility of Wernicke's aphasia in any patient who presents with an acute onset of a "confusional" state; listen carefully for the presence of paraphasic errors and neologisms that may help you determine that the "confused" patient is actually aphasic.
- Transcortical aphasias are additional types of aphasia that occur due to lesions near but not in Broca's area (transcortical motor aphasia) or Wernicke's area (transcortical sensory aphasia). The transcortical aphasias resemble Broca's or Wernicke's aphasias, but the ability to repeat is intact. These types of aphasia are not discussed further in this text because, for the purposes of gross neuroanatomic localization, it generally suffices to simply recognize that the patient has a motor or sensory aphasia and, therefore, likely has a problem in the dominant hemisphere that is most likely in or near the frontal lobe (motor aphasia) or the temporal lobe (sensory aphasia).

MEMORY TESTING

PURPOSE

The purpose of memory testing is to look for evidence of difficulty remembering that can occur from illnesses that affect cognition in general (such as dementing diseases) or from illnesses that affect memory alone (amnesic disorders).

WHEN TO TEST MEMORY

The ability of your patient to recall recent and distant events is often evident during your conversation with the patient while you are taking the history. You should formally test memory when there is a complaint by the patient or the patient's family of a problem with memory or any other cognitive difficulty, or when you suspect a disorder of memory or cognition from your conversation with the patient.

NEUROANATOMY OF MEMORY

Definitions of the various aspects of memory differ depending on whether you are talking to a clinical neurologist or a neuropsychologist. Most neurologists simply divide the kinds of memory that we test (called *episodic memory*) into immediate recall, short-term memory, and long-term memory, and the following discussion defines these terms as they are commonly used and understood by most clinical neurologists.

Immediate recall (also called *working memory*) refers to the kind of memory that we use to remember things for seconds, and it should probably be thought of more within the realm of concentration than memory. Examples of immediate recall include remembering a telephone number for the few seconds before finding a piece of paper on which to write it down or remembering the beginning of a sentence before getting to the end of the sentence. The neuroanatomic localization for immediate recall is not clear.

Short-term (also called *recent*) *memory* refers to memory for events that occurred minutes, days, weeks, or even months ago. Examples of short-term memories include remembering what you had for breakfast this morning or for dinner last Sunday, or where you went on vacation last month. The brain structures that are involved in the ability to recall short-term memories are the hippocampi (which reside in the medial temporal lobes) and the thalami.

Long-term memory refers to memory for distant events, such as events that occurred years ago. Examples of long-term memories include remembering where you lived and went to school when you were a child. Where these long-term memories reside within the brain is not clear, but they probably are stored somewhere within and possibly throughout the cerebral cortex.

EQUIPMENT NEEDED TO TEST MEMORY

None.

HOW TO EXAMINE MEMORY

Immediate Recall (Working Memory)

1. Tell the patient you will be asking him or her to repeat a list of numbers back to you after you have recited the list.

2. Recite a list of approximately six or seven single-digit numbers to the patient, such as "3, 9, 6, 4, 8, 7."
3. Listen to the patient's ability to repeat the numbers back to you and note any errors or omissions. Repeat the test with a shorter list if the patient has difficulties.
4. Another test of immediate recall—and probably all that is usually necessary to test this—is imbedded in the initial part of the short-term memory test: A patient's ability to immediately repeat three words back to you (that you give to test short-term memory as described below) is a test of immediate recall.

Short-Term (Recent) Memory

1. Tell the patient you will be asking him or her to try to remember three words that you will recite. Explain to the patient that you will ask him or her to repeat the words immediately to you and that you also want the patient to remember the words because you will ask him or her to recall the words again in a few minutes.
2. Tell the patient the three words. Choose simple but unrelated words; a common choice is "apple, table, penny," but any three words will do.
3. Ask the patient to repeat the words back to you. If the patient is able to immediately recall all the words, remind the patient that you will ask him or her to repeat the words back to you in a few minutes. If the patient is unable to immediately repeat all three words, restate the words until he or she is able to immediately recall all of them.
4. Wait approximately 2 minutes. During the intervening minutes, bide the small amount of time (e.g., make notes in your chart, talk with the patient, or perform another brief part of the examination).
5. Ask the patient what the three words were that you instructed him or her to remember. Make a note of any errors or omissions.
6. If the patient forgets one or some of the words, it is helpful to give the patient a clue (such as "One of the words was a kind of fruit") and see if this prods the patient into recalling the forgotten word.

Long-Term (Distant) Memory

1. Testing long-term memory is imbedded in taking the patient's history, such as when you ask about past medical illnesses, family history, and the patient's occupation. To specifically test the patient's recall of distant memories not already included in the routine history, ask the patient a verifiable question, such as where he or she grew up and where he or she went to high school or college.
2. Verify that the answer is correct by asking a family member if one is present with the patient. In the absence of such verification, accuracy of long-term memories may be difficult to confirm.

NORMAL FINDINGS
Immediate Recall

Normally, patients should be able to correctly immediately recall a list of approximately six numbers, and they should also be able to immediately recall the three words that you give them when you begin the test of short-term memory.

Short-Term (Recent) Memory

Patients should normally be able to recall three words after a delay of a few minutes. Note, though, that the ability to successfully recall a word or words with clues does suggest some intact memory for that word and can also be consistent with normal memory function (one way to report this finding on a memory test would be, "The patient recalled two out of three words after 2 minutes, and did recall the third word after given a clue.").

Long-Term (Distant) Memory

Normally, patients should be able to accurately recall significant personal events from the distant past.

ABNORMAL FINDINGS

Immediate Recall

- Difficulty correctly recalling a list of six numbers or difficulty immediately recalling the three words that you give the patient when you begin the test of short-term memory is consistent with difficulty in immediate recall.
- Because immediate recall is more of a test of concentration than memory, errors of immediate recall suggest difficulty with concentration and attention (see Chapter 8, Testing Orientation, Concentration, Knowledge, and Constructional Ability), as can be seen as a result of any cause of (diffuse or focal) brain dysfunction.

Short-Term (Recent) Memory

- Difficulty remembering any of three words, even with clues, after a few minutes suggests a problem with short-term memory.
- Problems with short-term memory suggest dysfunction of the hippocampal or medial thalamic memory structures. Generally, to have significant impairment of short-term memory, there needs to be bilateral dysfunction of these structures. For example, a unilateral hippocampal or medial thalamic lesion usually does not significantly affect short-term memory. Memory is usually severely affected by bilateral hippocampal or bilateral medial thalamic lesions, however. Such dysfunction of the hippocampal/thalamic memory system can be seen due to focal lesions affecting these areas alone (amnesic disorders) or, for example, as part of the diffuse cortical dysfunction that can be seen in dementing illnesses.

Long-Term (Distant) Memory

Problem with recall of significant distant personal events is unusual and would mainly be seen in the context of diffuse cortical dysfunction, such as can occur from severe dementing illnesses. In most cases of dementia, however, recall of past events is affected later and less severely than recent memories.

ADDITIONAL POINTS

- It is rare for patients to lose memory for self. Loss of personal identity suggests a nonneurologic cause of the "memory" dysfunction, such as conversion disorders or malingering.
- The kind of memory assessed in clinical neurology, as described in this chapter, is called *episodic memory*. Episodic memory refers to memory for events and experiences (including memory for a list of words presented by the examiner); it is episodic memory that we divide into time-related functions, such as immediate recall and short-term and long-term memories. Other types of memory function include procedural memory (memory for skills, such as how to ride a bicycle) and semantic memory (memory for facts, concepts, and the meaning of words). Unlike episodic memory, these types of memories are not related to specific events or experiences, and they are not what we're testing at the bedside when we examine memory in clinical neurology.

Chapter 8

TESTING ORIENTATION, CONCENTRATION, KNOWLEDGE, AND CONSTRUCTIONAL ABILITY

PURPOSE

The purpose of testing parameters of cognitive function is mainly to look for evidence of any diffuse or focal brain disorder that can affect cognition.

WHEN TO TEST ORIENTATION, CONCENTRATION, KNOWLEDGE, AND CONSTRUCTIONAL ABILITY

You should assess your patient's orientation, concentration, or knowledge whenever there is any clinical suspicion for or complaint of cognitive dysfunction. Testing constructional ability (e.g., clock drawing) is helpful whenever a disorder of cognition is suspected, but it is particularly useful if you suspect a focal right hemisphere process. None of these mental status tests need to be formally performed if there is no clinical suspicion or complaint of an abnormality of mental status or right hemispheric function.

NEUROANATOMY OF ORIENTATION, CONCENTRATION, KNOWLEDGE, AND CONSTRUCTIONAL ABILITY

Orientation, concentration, and knowledge are not clearly localizable to a specific neuroanatomic area of the brain and should be thought of as requiring the coordinated effort of multiple (diffuse) regions of the cerebral hemispheres. Constructional ability, however, resides primarily in the nondominant (usually right) hemisphere.

EQUIPMENT NEEDED TO TEST ORIENTATION, CONCENTRATION, KNOWLEDGE, AND CONSTRUCTIONAL ABILITY

Pen or pencil and paper.

HOW TO EXAMINE ORIENTATION, CONCENTRATION, KNOWLEDGE, AND CONSTRUCTIONAL ABILITY

Orientation

1. To assess if the patient is oriented to place, simply ask where he or she is. If the patient is able to respond correctly in a general way (e.g., in a hospital or in a clinic), try to see how specific his or her answer can be, such as which hospital room number or which floor of the clinic. If he or she is unable to respond to the general question correctly, ask an even more general question, such as what city he or she is in.
2. To assess if the patient is oriented to time, simply ask what the date is (including the month, date, year, and the day of the week). If you suspect

the patient may have difficulty knowing the exact date, start the questioning more generally by asking what year it is before asking more specifically about the month, day of the week, and date.

Concentration

Concentration is tested by asking the patient to perform a task that requires juggling of information in the patient's mind, and, therefore, these tasks need to be performed without the patient using pencil or paper. In practice, concentration is often tested by asking the patient to spell a word (such as "world") backward, after showing that he or she can correctly spell it forward. Another test of concentration is the test of *serial sevens*. To test serial sevens, ask the patient to "subtract seven from one hundred and then keep going down by sevens," with the patient reciting the answers one by one aloud. Avoid the serial seven test if the patient's educational status suggests that the calculation involved (which is not trivial if the patient has only a partial grammar school education) would be a problem.

Knowledge

Knowledge can be assessed in many ways, including asking about personal information (e.g., "How many grandchildren do you have?") or about current events (e.g., "Who's the President of the United States?" or "What's going on in the news these days?"). To save time, it's probably best to start with a more difficult question and proceed to easier questions if the patient has problems with the harder ones.

Constructional Ability

Constructional ability can be tested in several ways. One useful test for constructional ability consists of asking the patient to draw a clock. To do so, draw a circle on a piece of paper, making sure that the circle is big enough (e.g., more than 2 in. in diameter) that the patient can comfortably fill in the numbers, and then ask the patient to "Draw the numbers of a clock in the circle." Once the patient has filled in the numbers, ask the patient to draw the hands to make the clock read a particular time (e.g., "Draw the hands of the clock to make the clock read 2:30.").

Clinicians also often test constructional ability by asking the patient to copy a diagram showing two pentagons intersecting at one corner (so that a four-sided figure is created by the intersecting sides); this is the constructional task included within the commonly performed Mini-Mental State Examination (see Chapter 5, Approach to the Mental Status Examination).

NORMAL FINDINGS

Orientation

Normally, patients should be oriented to place (including the name of the hospital or clinic and the floor of the building) and time (including day of the week, date, month, and year).

Concentration

Normally, patients should be able to spell the word "world" backward if they can correctly spell it forward. Assuming a baseline ability to subtract appropriately, patients should be able to perform serial sevens down to the 50s or 60s.

Knowledge

Patients should normally be able to give you correct personal information, such as their address and the number of children and grandchildren they have. Patients should also have knowledge of current events compatible with their baseline level of education and interest.

Constructional Ability

Patients should be able to draw all of the numbers of a clock in the approximate correct places, should not ignore any side of the clock, and should be able to place the clock hands in the appropriate places. Patients should also be able to copy a figure, such as two intersecting pentagons, keeping both figures five-sided, and they should be able to correctly copy the intersection of the two pentagons as a four-sided figure.

ABNORMAL FINDINGS

Orientation

Disorientation to place or time is abnormal and consistent with any abnormality of cognition. This is not localizable to a specific hemispheric region and is most suggestive of diffuse or multifocal brain dysfunction.

Concentration

Abnormalities on tests for concentration include difficulties spelling the word "world" backward or errors performing serial sevens (assuming the patient has the baseline ability to subtract). Difficulties with concentration are not localizable to a particular hemispheric region and can be seen due to any cause of diffuse or multifocal brain dysfunction.

Knowledge

Lack of knowledge of personal information, such as home address or information about family members, is usually clearly abnormal. Be careful, though, not to overinterpret gaps in knowledge of current events or knowledge of public figures (such as the name of the President or especially the Vice President), unless it is clear that this information would have been known at baseline. Abnormalities of knowledge should always be interpreted within the context of your presumption of the patient's baseline level of cognitive functioning (based on the history you have obtained from the patient or family) and should be considered indicative of a new abnormality only if worse than baseline. Most abnormalities of knowledge are not localizable to a particular hemispheric region and can be seen due to any cause of diffuse or multifocal brain dysfunction. Recently acquired knowledge, however, may be lost due to deficits in short-term memory, such as can be due to bilateral temporal lobe dysfunction, as described in Chapter 7, Memory Testing.

Constructional Ability

- Errors in clock drawing can include incorrect placement of numbers, repeating numbers, and incorrect placement of the clock hands. Errors in drawing the intersecting pentagons include any errors in drawing the correct number of sides or the appropriate intersection of the two figures. Although all these errors in constructional ability suggest the possibility of focal nondominant (usually right) parietal pathology, most of these errors are nonspecific and can also be seen as a result of any diffuse or multifocal hemispheric dysfunction.
- A more specific and localizing kind of error can be seen when testing constructional ability. Patients who consistently leave out the left side of the clock (i.e., drawing all of the numbers on the right side) or ignore the left

side of a figure when copying it have evidence for left-sided neglect that is suggestive of a focal nondominant (right) parietal cortical process.

ADDITIONAL POINTS

- Assessment of other aspects of cognition, such as abstract thinking or judgment, can sometimes be useful. These tests may be helpful, for example, when a frontal lobe dementia is suspected, because memory and other aspects of cognition that are routinely tested may not be abnormal early in this condition.
  - To test abstract thinking, ask the patient to interpret a proverb (one you would assume the patient would have heard), such as "A stitch in time saves nine." Don't look for perfection; simply listen for significant abnormalities, such as extreme concreteness or any unusual response.
  - One way to test judgment is to ask what the patient would do if he or she found a stamped, sealed, addressed envelope on the ground. There is no single correct answer to this scenario, but listen for the general appropriateness of the response.
- All the tests of cognitive function described in this chapter (as well as the tests described in Chapter 7, Memory Testing) would be significantly affected if language function is abnormal (see Chapter 6, Language Testing) and, therefore, are difficult to perform and interpret in the presence of aphasias, especially Wernicke's aphasia.
- As described in Chapter 7, Memory Testing, knowledge for self is rarely lost, even in patients with a severe lack of orientation to place and time, and it usually does not need to be specifically asked when testing orientation. The loss of personal identity in an awake, communicative (nonaphasic) patient suggests a nonneurologic cause of that dysfunction.

Chapter 9

APPROACH TO THE EXAMINATION OF THE CRANIAL NERVES

PURPOSE

The purpose of the examination of the cranial nerves is to localize neurologic disease by looking for evidence of cranial nerve dysfunction that can occur due to disorders of the brain, brainstem, or cranial nerves themselves.

WHEN TO EXAMINE THE CRANIAL NERVES

Assessment of the most diagnostically relevant cranial nerve functions should be performed on all patients as part of any standard neurologic examination. The examination elements that should be checked routinely, the elements that usually can be skipped, and the elements that need only be performed when specific clinical questions are being asked are explained in subsequent chapters of this section and summarized in Chapter 40, Performing a Complete Neurologic Examination.

NEUROANATOMY OF THE CRANIAL NERVES

All of the cranial nerves, with the exception of the first (olfactory) and second (optic) nerves, have nuclei within the brainstem and exit the brainstem to innervate their motor or sensory structures (or both) in the head. The first and second nerves are different than the others in that they are best thought of as extensions of the brain; the optic nerves actually are central nervous system structures.

EQUIPMENT NEEDED TO EXAMINE THE CRANIAL NERVES

- A bright flashlight
- An ophthalmoscope
- A pocket-sized eye chart card
- A safety pin and a cotton swab
- A 512-Hz tuning fork
- A tongue depressor and a flashlight

HOW TO EXAMINE THE CRANIAL NERVES

The specifics of examining cranial nerve function are described in subsequent chapters of this section. These chapters are not categorized by individual cranial nerves; instead, each chapter describes a functional examination element. For example, there is no chapter labeled "Examination of the Third Cranial Nerve." Instead, the assessment of function of the ophthalmic nerve is imbedded within Chapter 14, Examination of Eye Movements, and Chapter 10, Examination of the Pupils, because these are the clinical tests that provide information about the function of this nerve.

NORMAL FINDINGS

Normally, patients should have intact motor or sensory function, or both, of each of the cranial nerves.

ABNORMAL FINDINGS

Cranial nerve dysfunction is manifested on examination by weakness of the muscle(s) that the cranial nerve innervates or by loss of sensory function in the distribution of the nerve. Chapters 9 through 23 describe the most common clinically relevant abnormal findings on cranial nerve testing, explain which cranial nerve abnormalities cause these findings, and address the potential diagnostic implications.

ADDITIONAL POINTS

Try to approach your examination of the cranial nerves by function, in the same manner that the following chapters in this section are presented. Organize your cranial nerve examination by functional components (e.g., pupillary function, eye movements, facial strength) and then decide which of the cranial nerves is responsible for any abnormal findings you detect on examination. Rote examination of individual cranial nerves one by one is complicated and inefficient.

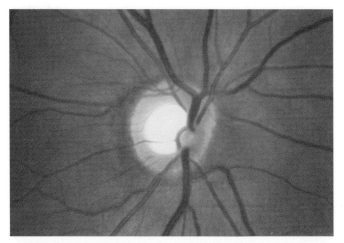

Figure 11-1 A normal optic disc.

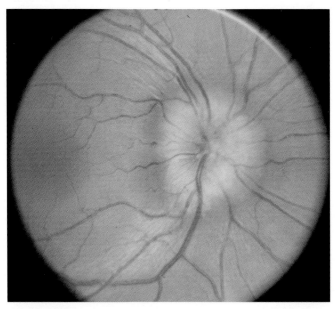

Figure 11-2 An optic disc with severe papilledema.

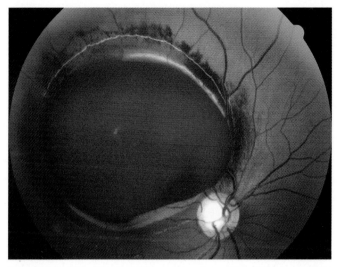

Figure 11–3 Retinal (subhyaloid) hemorrhage in a patient with a subarachnoid hemorrhage.

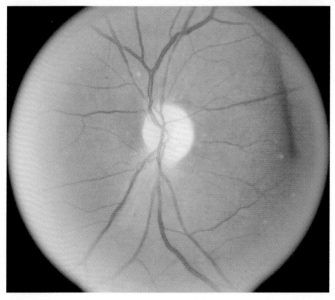

Figure 11–4 Optic atrophy in a patient with severe chronic optic nerve dysfunction.

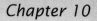

Chapter 10

EXAMINATION OF THE PUPILS

PURPOSE

Examination of Resting Pupillary Size and Symmetry and the Pupillary Response to Light

The purpose of the assessment of pupillary size and symmetry and the pupillary light reaction is to provide information regarding the efferent pathways that constrict and dilate the pupils, as well as the afferent pathways through which light is transmitted in the optic nerves.

Examination of the Pupillary Response to Near

The purpose of examining the pupillary response to near is to assess for the presence of rare disorders that impair the ability of the pupil to constrict to light but spare the ability of the pupil to constrict when focusing on a close object.

Examination for an Afferent Pupillary Defect (the Swinging Flashlight Test)

The purpose of testing for an afferent pupillary defect is to look for any significant asymmetry of optic nerve function of one side compared to the other.

WHEN TO PERFORM THE DIFFERENT COMPONENTS OF THE PUPILLARY EXAMINATION

Examination of Resting Pupillary Size and Symmetry

Observation of resting pupillary size and side-to-side symmetry should be performed on all patients as part of a standard neurologic examination.

Examination of the Pupillary Response to Light

Testing for the pupillary light reaction should be performed on all patients as part of a standard neurologic examination.

Examination of the Pupillary Response to Near

Testing for pupillary constriction to near needs to be performed only when there is an obviously absent or extremely slow pupillary light reaction, either unilaterally or bilaterally. There is no need to check for pupillary constriction to near if normal constriction to light is already demonstrated, because there is no clinically important condition that affects pupillary constriction to a near stimulus alone.

Examination for an Afferent Pupillary Defect (the Swinging Flashlight Test)

Testing for an afferent pupillary defect needs to be performed only when there is a clinical complaint (or evidence) of unilateral visual dysfunction or a history suggestive of a previous episode of significant visual dysfunction affecting one eye more than the other. Without a history of significant asymmetric vision loss, there is no need to test for an afferent pupillary defect.

33

NEUROANATOMY OF PUPILLARY FUNCTION

Resting Pupillary Size and Symmetry

Resting pupillary size is determined by the balance between the parasympathetic efferent pathways that constrict the pupils and the sympathetic efferent pathways that dilate the pupils. Symmetry of pupillary size occurs because of the reflex pathways that mediate the bilateral consensual pupillary constriction to light described in the following section, Pupillary Response to Light.

Pupillary Response to Light

Pupillary constriction to light is a reflex mediated afferently by visual pathways that begin in each retina and travel in each optic nerve. After crossing in the optic chiasm, reflex fibers from each eye project to the midbrain and bilaterally innervate the Edinger-Westphal nuclei, components of the third nerve nuclei. Efferent fibers from each Edinger-Westphal nucleus travel with the third cranial nerve, synapse in the parasympathetic ciliary ganglion, and cause contraction of the muscles that constrict the pupil. Because of the bilateral reflex innervation to the Edinger-Westphal nuclei, light shined on one eye should cause constriction of that eye (the direct response) and also cause constriction of the opposite eye (the consensual response).

Pupillary Response to Near

When attempting to focus on a close object, a reflex occurs that results in bilateral pupillary constriction mediated efferently by parasympathetic fibers from the ciliary ganglion. This pupillary constriction to near (which can be seen clinically) accompanies the reflex thickening of the lens, called *accommodation* (which cannot be assessed clinically), that occurs due to contraction of the ciliary muscles that are also innervated by the ciliary ganglion.

Afferent Pupillary Defect

The neuroanatomy of an afferent pupillary defect is described in the section Abnormal Findings.

EQUIPMENT NEEDED TO EXAMINE THE PUPILS

- A bright flashlight
- The cheap, disposable flashlights common in hospital settings are good when brand new, but they quickly become dim and of little value for the pupillary examination. More expensive flashlights with replaceable batteries are reasonable alternatives, as long as they can be focused into a beam that can reliably constrict normal pupils. The light of a rechargeable otoscope is a good source of light for the pupillary examination.

HOW TO EXAMINE THE PUPILS

Examination of Resting Pupillary Size and Symmetry

1. Ask the patient to look straight ahead at a distant spot in a dim room. It is helpful to show the patient a specific spot on the wall (or the ceiling, if the patient is lying down) to fixate on.
2. Look at the resting position of both pupils. Note whether both pupils are approximately the same size or whether there is any obvious difference in pupillary size. If necessary (especially if there is a difference in size between sides), pupillary diameter can be measured with a ruler or the pupillary size chart found on most pocket visual acuity cards.

Examination of the Pupillary Response to Light

1. Ask the patient to look straight ahead at a distant spot in a dim room.
2. Shine a bright light in one eye. Shine the light from the lateral side of the eye or from beneath to help ensure that the patient doesn't accommodate to a near stimulus during the assessment of pupillary light reaction. Assess whether the pupil constricts to the light stimulus.
3. After removing the light stimulus and waiting a few seconds, move the light to the other eye and assess whether that pupil constricts to light.

Examination of the Pupillary Response to Near

1. In a well-lit room (so that you can see the pupils without shining a light into them), ask the patient to fixate on a distant spot directly ahead, such as a spot on the wall. Note the pupillary size while the patient fixates on that spot.
2. Next, ask the patient to look down at his or her nose. If the patient has difficulty with this maneuver, an alternative near stimulus is to have the patient look at an object, such as your finger or a pen, held within inches in front of the eyes.
3. Observe for pupillary constriction while the patient focuses on this near stimulus for at least several seconds.

Examination for an Afferent Pupillary Defect (the Swinging Flashlight Test)

1. Assess the pupillary light reaction of one pupil as described above. After that pupil constricts, immediately move the flashlight over to the other eye and assess the reaction of the other pupil (constriction or dilatation) to direct light. The light should be kept on each pupil for approximately 1 to 2 seconds before moving the flashlight over to the other eye.
2. Next, move the flashlight back to the original eye and assess its response to direct light.
3. Repeat the process of moving the flashlight from eye to eye a few times while you confirm the response of each pupil after the light has been moved to that eye.

NORMAL FINDINGS

Examination of Resting Pupillary Size and Symmetry

Normally, the pupils should be approximately equal in size.

Examination of the Pupillary Response to Light

Normally, each pupil should constrict when a light is shined directly into it (the direct pupillary response), and each pupil should constrict when a light is shined into the contralateral pupil (the consensual pupillary response).

Examination of the Pupillary Response to Near

Normally, the pupils should both constrict when focusing on a near object.

Examination for an Afferent Pupillary Defect (the Swinging Flashlight Test)

Normally, each pupil should constrict or stay the same size when the light is moved to it from the other eye.

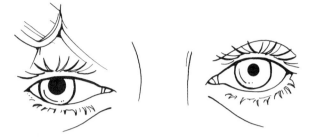

Figure 10–1 Unilateral pupillary dilatation due to a third cranial nerve palsy. The pupil does not react to light, and in this case, the ptosis is so severe that the examiner needs to lift the patient's eyelid to examine the eye. There is also lateral and downward deviation of the eye because of the weakness of third nerve–innervated extraocular muscles.

ABNORMAL FINDINGS

Examination of Resting Pupillary Size and Symmetry

- Asymmetry of the size of the pupils (anisocoria) may be seen when there is any lesion of the efferent pathways that constrict or dilate the pupil. When anisocoria is present, it is not always immediately obvious as to which pupil is the abnormally large or small one, but certain clues (see below) usually help determine this.
- As long as the pupils are approximately equal in size bilaterally, the absolute size of the pupils—whether bilaterally small or large—is usually of no clinical significance in awake patients. In comatose patients, however, pupillary size, even when symmetric, may have significant diagnostic value, as discussed in Chapter 42, Examination of the Comatose Patient.

Examination of the Pupillary Response to Light

- A unilaterally enlarged (dilated) pupil that reacts poorly or not at all to light suggests a lesion of the pupillary constricting fibers of the ipsilateral third cranial nerve. Although pupillary dilatation may be the only sign of a third nerve palsy, other clues include ptosis on the side of the dilated pupil and weakness of adduction, upward, and downward movement of the eye. Figure 10–1 illustrates a patient with unilateral pupillary dilatation due to a third cranial nerve palsy.
- A unilaterally small (constricted or miotic) but reactive pupil suggests a lesion anywhere along the ipsilateral sympathetic pathway that normally dilates the eye (Horner's syndrome). In addition to miosis, other findings of Horner's syndrome may also be present, including slight ptosis and diminished sweating on the same side of the face as the small pupil. Figure 10–2 illustrates a patient with a unilateral miotic pupil due to Horner's syndrome.
- Complete absence of a direct pupillary response to light on one side with retention of the consensual response of that pupil when light is shined in the other eye is most consistent with severe optic nerve dysfunction on the side of the absent direct response. This is the ultimate afferent pupillary defect (see below).

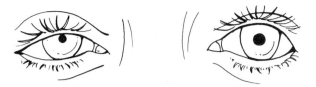

Figure 10–2 Unilateral pupillary constriction (miosis) due to Horner's syndrome. The pupil is small, reacts to light, and there is slight ptosis on the side of the miotic pupil.

Examination of the Pupillary Response to Near

- A pupil with an absent reaction to light but normal constriction to near is called a *light-near dissociated pupil.*
- Light-near dissociated pupils are found in relatively rare conditions, such as Adie's pupil syndrome, Argyll Robertson pupil of neurosyphilis, or lesions of the pineal region (the dorsal midbrain/thalamic region).

Examination for an Afferent Pupillary Defect (the Swinging Flashlight Test)

- The finding of immediate pupillary dilation—rather than constriction or no change in size—when the light is moved to it is consistent with an afferent pupillary defect (also known as a *Marcus Gunn pupil*) on that side.
- The finding of an afferent pupillary defect implies significant relative dysfunction of the afferent visual pathway anterior to the optic chiasm (most likely the optic nerve) of that eye compared to the other eye.
- The clinical finding of an afferent pupillary defect occurs because the pupil on the side of the abnormal optic nerve retains its ability to constrict to a light shined in the contralateral eye due to the intact efferent pathways of the consensual pupillary reflex. When a light is moved from the good eye and then shined in the affected eye, however, dilatation occurs because the direct response through the abnormal side is a weaker stimulus than the constriction that occurred from the consensual response.

ADDITIONAL POINTS

Examination of Resting Pupillary Size and Symmetry

- Small, side-to-side differences in pupillary size (e.g., approximately 1 mm) may be physiologic (called *physiologic anisocoria*).
- Lesions involving the visual afferent pathways anterior to the optic chiasm (the retina or the optic nerves) do not cause anisocoria, because of the bilateral innervation of the reflex mechanism for consensual pupillary constriction.
- Lesions of the visual pathways posterior to the optic chiasm also do not affect resting pupillary size or symmetry.

Examination of the Pupillary Response to Light

Lesions of the afferent visual pathways posterior to the optic chiasm do not affect the pupillary response to light, because the pathways for the pupillary light reaction occur anterior to the chiasm.

Examination of the Pupillary Response to Near

Although it is not necessary to test for pupillary constriction to near except in cases in which there is an abnormal pupillary light reaction, it is useful to practice this test in patients with normal pupillary light responses so that you will be adept at performing this examination when it is clinically appropriate.

Examination for an Afferent Pupillary Defect (the Swinging Flashlight Test)

- Afferent pupillary defects are most obvious when the patient has severe unilateral vision loss due to an optic nerve lesion, such as from optic neuritis.
- By definition, it is impossible to have bilateral afferent pupillary defects!
- Do not confuse hippus (common mild waxing and waning variations in pupillary size) with an afferent pupillary defect.
- Patients with afferent pupillary defects do not have anisocoria because of the presence of normal bilateral reflex mechanisms for efferent pupillary constriction (see above).

Chapter 11

FUNDUSCOPIC EXAMINATION

PURPOSE

The main purpose of optic funduscopy in the neurologic examination is to look for swelling of the optic disc. In the clinical context in which subarachnoid hemorrhage is a consideration, another purpose of funduscopy is to look for retinal hemorrhages.

WHEN TO PERFORM THE FUNDUSCOPIC EXAMINATION

An attempt at visualization of the optic fundus should be performed on all patients as part of a standard neurologic examination.

NEUROANATOMY OF THE FUNDUSCOPIC EXAMINATION

The optic nerves are formed from the axons of retinal neurons that converge to exit the eye and send visual information back to the brain. The optic disc, also called the *optic nerve head*, is the portion of the optic nerve that can be visualized when looking in the optic fundus. The optic discs are located in a slightly medial position within the retina; this is important to remember when trying to visualize the optic disc.

The subarachnoid space that surrounds the brain and spinal cord also extends into the optic nerves. Therefore, processes that increase the intracranial pressure can also extend their pressure along the optic nerves, which may be visualized as swelling of the optic nerve head (papilledema).

EQUIPMENT NEEDED FOR THE FUNDUSCOPIC EXAMINATION

An ophthalmoscope.

HOW TO EXAMINE THE OPTIC FUNDUS

1. Begin by preparing the ophthalmoscope. Set the ophthalmoscope to 0 diopters, the optimal initial setting for most patients and physicians. Set the light of the ophthalmoscope so that it produces a white circle of light.
2. Ask the patient to look straight ahead at a distant spot in a dim room. It is helpful to show the patient a specific spot on the wall in front of the patient to fixate on (or a spot on the ceiling if the patient is lying in bed). Being in a dim room, rather than a dark room, better allows the patient to see the spot and helps with fixation. Ask the patient to try to keep fixating on that spot without moving his or her eyes.
3. Hold the ophthalmoscope to your eye. Look through the ophthalmoscope with your right eye to assess the patient's right eye, and look through the ophthalmoscope with your left eye to examine the patient's left eye.
4. While holding the ophthalmoscope to your eye and shining it into your patient's pupil, bring the ophthalmoscope in from the temporal side of the eye so that you are aiming slightly toward the medial side of the retina.

5. Bring the ophthalmoscope in toward the patient as you continue to try to visualize the optic disc. Generally by this time you should be close to the patient. To avoid striking the patient's eye with the ophthalmoscope, it is helpful to hold your index finger slightly outward so that this rests against the patient's cheek, using your other fingers to grip the ophthalmoscope tightly.

6. Adjust the lens in the positive (black) or negative (red) direction, if needed, to bring the optic disc into focus.

NORMAL FINDINGS

Normally, the optic discs should be sharp, with reasonably well-defined margins, and have a yellowish-orange color (Fig. 11–1). There should be no hemorrhages in the retina.

ABNORMAL FINDINGS

Optic Disc Swelling

- Mild swelling of the optic disc is manifested by obliteration of the usually sharp disc margins. Severe swelling of the optic disc is manifested by severe edema and obliteration of the disc margins (Fig. 11–2); there may also be hemorrhages around the swollen disc.

- Swelling of the optic disc can be due to increased intracranial pressure (papilledema) or inflammation of the optic disc (papillitis). These two major causes of optic disc swelling cannot be differentiated through ophthalmoscopy alone. It is a useful general rule, however, that acute papilledema does not cause any significant effect on visual acuity, whereas papillitis causes vision loss. Papilledema does, however, cause enlargement of the physiologic blind spot on visual field testing, and chronic papilledema can cause vision loss.

Retinal Hemorrhages

Hemorrhages in the retina (subhyaloid hemorrhages) can be seen in some patients with subarachnoid hemorrhage (Fig. 11–3).

Optic Atrophy

Optic nerve head atrophy is manifested by severe pallor (whiteness) of the optic disc (Fig. 11–4). Optic atrophy is seen when there is severe chronic optic nerve dysfunction.

ADDITIONAL POINTS

- Becoming comfortable with ophthalmoscopy to visualize the optic discs requires practice, but it is not really difficult.

- It is not reasonable for a nonophthalmologist to be expected to be adept at recognizing subtle vascular or retinal changes. Concentrate on what you really need to be able to assess in the neurologic examination: the optic disc. The more normal optic discs you evaluate, the more likely that you will recognize an abnormally swollen one.

- It is not usually necessary to use mydriatic agents (eyedrops that dilate the pupil) to visualize the optic disc to assess for disc swelling in the routine neurologic examination. Some patients have small pupils that make visualization of the optic discs difficult, however. When the optic discs cannot be visualized and the clinical situation particularly warrants the examination of the discs to rule out papilledema or hemorrhages, mydriatic agents can be considered.

Chapter 12

EXAMINATION OF VISUAL ACUITY

PURPOSE

The main purpose of the examination of visual acuity during the neurologic examination is to determine how well the optic nerves are functioning.

WHEN TO TEST VISUAL ACUITY

Visual acuity should be assessed during the neurologic examination if the patient has any visual symptoms or if the patient is thought to have a condition that can ultimately affect vision. In the absence of these situations, it is not imperative to check visual acuity in all patients as part of a routine neurologic examination.

NEUROANATOMY OF VISUAL ACUITY

Visual acuity of each eye depends on the integrity of the eye (anterior compartment and posterior compartment, including the retina) and the optic nerve. Lesions posterior to the optic chiasm affect visual fields (see Chapter 13, Visual Field Examination) but do not cause abnormal visual acuity within the intact fields.

EQUIPMENT NEEDED TO TEST VISUAL ACUITY

A pocket-sized eye chart card used to determine reading vision (also called a *near card*).

HOW TO EXAMINE VISUAL ACUITY

1. In a brightly lit room, have the patient hold the visual acuity card in one hand, while using the other hand to keep one eye closed. If the patient needs visual correction for reading, have the patient use this.
2. Have the patient hold the card approximately 14 in. away. (Holding the card at a specific, exact, distance is not imperative from the standpoint of the neurologic examination. Have the patient hold the card at a reasonably comfortable distance, which usually ends up being approximately 14 in. away anyway.)
3. Point to the 20/20 line on the card and ask the patient to read the numbers. If the patient is unable to read the 20/20 line, point to the next higher line until the patient is able to read most of the numbers correctly. Report this line as the visual acuity.
4. Repeat with the other eye.

NORMAL FINDINGS

With the appropriate refractive correction for reading, most patients with normal optic nerve function should have close to 20/20 vision in each eye.

ABNORMAL FINDINGS

- The abnormal finding on visual acuity testing is diminished visual acuity. Depending on the clinical situation, a visual acuity of 20/25 or worse can be considered abnormal, as long as the acuity is tested with the patient wearing the appropriate refractive correction.

- Visual acuity can be affected by dysfunction of the eye or the optic nerve. The finding of abnormal visual acuity despite appropriate refractive correction suggests optic nerve dysfunction, because most patients with normal optic nerve function can be corrected with the appropriate lenses to nearly 20/20 for reading. Other ophthalmologic (e.g., retinal) causes of diminished visual acuity may need to be excluded through ophthalmologic consultation, however.

ADDITIONAL POINTS

- Patients sometimes need coaxing to read the smallest line that represents their true acuity.
- It often helps to shine a bright light on the card to improve brightness and contrast, allowing demonstration of the best visual acuity.
- If the patient normally uses reading glasses but does not have them available, the patient's near vision can be tested through a pinhole. A pinhole acts like a lens that corrects the refractive error for near vision of most patients (who have normal optic nerve function) to close to 20/20, albeit within a small field of vision. A pinhole can be created on the spot by taking a small piece of cardboard and making a hole in it with a safety pin. The patient should be asked to hold this up to each eye and to read the card through the hole. Try this on yourself (especially if you need correction for reading) and see how well it works.

Chapter 13

VISUAL FIELD EXAMINATION

PURPOSE

The purpose of the visual field examination is to assess the function of the visual pathway that begins in the eyes and ends in the occipital cortex, because lesions located along different regions of this pathway produce characteristic visual field abnormalities.

WHEN TO EXAMINE THE VISUAL FIELDS

Confrontational visual field testing is a quick and easy way of discovering significant visual field loss, and it should be performed on all patients as part of a standard neurologic examination.

NEUROANATOMY OF THE VISUAL FIELDS

The visual pathway is pictured in Figure 13–1. The nasal (medial) part of each retina sees the temporal visual world, and the temporal (lateral) part of each retina sees the nasal visual world. Visual information from each retina travels through the optic nerves into the optic chiasm. At the optic chiasm, the visual information from the nasal part of each retina crosses to the other side and continues as the optic tract, whereas the visual information from the lateral part of each retina remains uncrossed, also continuing as the optic tract. Each optic tract synapses in the lateral geniculate nucleus. From the lateral geniculate nuclei, the visual information continues onward toward the occipital cortex as the optic radiations. Visual information from the lower retina (which sees the upper fields) travels through the optic radiations that are located in the temporal lobes, reaching the lower occipital cortex. Visual information from the upper retina (which sees the lower fields) travels through the optic radiations that are located in the parietal lobes, reaching the upper part of the occipital cortex.

EQUIPMENT NEEDED FOR THE VISUAL FIELD EXAMINATION

None.

HOW TO EXAMINE THE VISUAL FIELDS

1. Stand a few feet in front of the patient, with your head at approximately the same level as the patient, looking directly at the patient's eyes.
2. Instruct the patient to look at your nose throughout the examination, and have the patient cover one eye with his or her hand. Ask the patient to count the total number of fingers you'll be holding up.
3. Check the visual fields by holding up one, two, or five fingers in the vertical plane that is just between you and the patient, checking each of the four quadrants. Test at least four separate areas: the left and right upper visual fields and the left and right lower visual fields. You do not need to hold the hands far into the periphery, only approximately 1 ft away from the midline. In most cases, you can quickly check both upper fields at the same time (for example, by holding up one finger with your left hand and

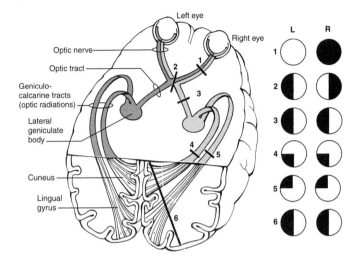

Figure 13-1 Illustration of the visual pathway from the eyes to the occipital cortex. The characteristic visual field deficits that would occur due to each of the numbered lesions at various regions of the visual pathway are shown. See text for further details. (Redrawn from Gilman S, Newman SW. Vision. In: *Manter and Gatz's essentials of clinical neuroanatomy and neurophysiology*, 8th ed. Philadelphia: FA Davis Co, 1992:196.)

two fingers with your right hand, asking the patient to tell you the total number of fingers you're holding up), and then examine both lower fields at the same time. If this is confusing to the patient, check each quadrant separately.

4. Repeat the same process with the patient's other eye closed.

NORMAL FINDINGS

Normally, patients should be able to count fingers in all visual fields of each eye: the left upper quadrant, left lower quadrant, right upper quadrant, and right lower quadrant.

ABNORMAL FINDINGS

- An inability to count fingers in a visual field, or visual fields, is abnormal.
- Visual field defects can occur from dysfunction of the visual pathway anywhere from the eyes to the occipital cortex. The typical visual field deficits that occur due to lesions at different regions of the visual pathway are illustrated in Figure 13-1 and discussed below.
- Visual fields are characteristically charted by drawing a circle representing the visual field of the left eye and another circle representing the visual field of the right eye. These are drawn as if you are the patient looking out: The left eye field is drawn on the left and the right eye field is drawn on the right. Intact visual fields are drawn as empty circles. Any abnormality of a visual field is indicated by filling in that portion of the

circle. Therefore, a patient with difficulty seeing in the left visual field of both eyes would be drawn as shown for lesion 3 of Figure 13–1.

- Visual field deficits that involve one eye only are called *monocular defects* and occur due to dysfunction anterior to the optic chiasm, such as the optic nerve. Lesion 1 of Figure 13–1 shows a lesion of the right optic nerve causing right eye (i.e., monocular) blindness.

- Bilateral temporal visual field defects (bitemporal hemianopsias) occur from lesions at the optic chiasm, due to dysfunction of the crossing fibers that arise from the nasal aspects of each retina. Lesion 2 of Figure 13–1 shows a lesion at the optic chiasm causing a bitemporal hemianopsia.

- Visual field deficits that involve the same visual field of both eyes are called *homonymous visual field defects* and are due to lesions posterior to the optic chiasm. Homonymous visual field defects can involve one entire side of each eye (right or left homonymous hemianopsias) or just the upper or lower quadrant (right or left upper or lower quadrantanopsias).

- Homonymous visual field defects involving an entire field (left or right homonymous hemianopsias) can arise due to a lesion of the optic tract, both the upper and lower optic radiations, or the occipital cortex. Lesion 3 of Figure 13–1 shows a left homonymous hemianopsia due to a lesion of the right optic tract. Lesion 6 of Figure 13–1 shows a left homonymous hemianopsia due to a lesion of the right occipital cortex.

- Homonymous quadrantanopsias occur due to a lesion involving one of the (upper or lower) optic radiations or a lesion involving just the upper or the lower part of the occipital cortex. Lesion 4 of Figure 13–1 shows a left lower quadrantanopsia due to a lesion of the right parietal optic radiations, and lesion 5 shows a left upper quadrantanopsia due to a lesion of the right temporal optic radiations.

ADDITIONAL POINTS

- Despite its simplicity and the rapidity with which it can be performed, confrontational visual field testing is a sensitive screening test that can detect significant visual field abnormalities produced by brain or optic nerve lesions.

- It is optimal to perform confrontational visual field testing of each eye individually, especially so that monocular field defects can be detected. For an even more rapid screening test of a patient who has no visual symptoms, however, it is occasionally reasonable to cheat by performing confrontational visual field testing with both of the patient's eyes open, although this would not exclude monocular defects.

- Patients with nondominant (usually right) hemisphere lesions may exhibit a phenomenon known as *visual field extinction*, also called *extinction on double-simultaneous stimulation*. These patients may have normal visual fields when asked to count fingers in the left or right fields separately, but they may ignore the left-sided stimuli when fingers are held up in both fields simultaneously. This finding is particularly suggestive of a right parietal lesion and is discussed further in Chapter 31, Examination of Cortical Sensation.

Chapter 14

EXAMINATION OF EYE MOVEMENTS

PURPOSE

The main purpose of the examination of eye movements is to look for evidence of dysfunction of the third or sixth cranial nerves, the extraocular muscles, or the brainstem. Another purpose of the eye movement examination is to assess the function of the central nervous system pathways that control voluntary conjugate gaze of the eyes.

WHEN TO TEST EYE MOVEMENTS

Eye movements should be examined in all patients as part of a standard neurologic examination.

NEUROANATOMY OF EYE MOVEMENTS

Cranial Nerves and Extraocular Muscles

The movements of each eye are directly due to the action of the six extraocular muscles that attach to the globe. Innervation to these extraocular muscles comes from three cranial nerves: the oculomotor (third) nerve, the abducens (sixth) nerve, and the trochlear (fourth) nerve. Table 14–1 summarizes the cranial nerve innervation to the extraocular muscles and the principal action of each muscle.

Central Nervous System Pathways for Voluntary Control of Gaze

Voluntary control of gaze occurs because of pathways that arise in the cerebral hemispheres and descend into the brainstem, ultimately controlling conjugate gaze through their action on the cranial nerve nuclei in the brainstem. Horizontal gaze (the most clinically important pathway to know about) is initiated by impulses from the "frontal eye field" of each cerebral hemisphere that project to the contralateral pons.

EQUIPMENT NEEDED TO EXAMINE EYE MOVEMENTS

None.

HOW TO EXAMINE EYE MOVEMENTS

1. Stand in front of the patient, holding your index finger approximately 1 ft or more away from the patient, holding the finger up vertically, midline between the patient's eyes.
2. Ask the patient to follow your finger with his or her eyes while keeping his or her head still. It sometimes helps to hold the patient's head still by gently resting your other hand on the patient's head or under the patient's chin.
3. Smoothly move your finger across to your right to observe the patient's horizontal eye movements toward the left.
4. Then smoothly move your finger across to your left to observe the patient's horizontal eye movements toward the right.

TABLE 14–1 Summary of the Innervation and Principal Actions of the Extraocular Muscles

Cranial Nerve	Origin of Cranial Nerve	Extraocular Muscles Innervated	Principal Action of Muscle
III (Oculomotor)	Midbrain	Superior rectus	Moves eye up
		Inferior rectus	Moves eye down
		Medial rectus	Moves eye medially
		Inferior oblique	Moves eye up (best when eye is in adducted position)
IV (Trochlear)	Midbrain	Superior oblique	Moves eye down (best when eye is in adducted position)
VI (Abducens)	Pons	Lateral rectus	Moves eye laterally

5. Move your finger back to the midline so that the patient's eyes follow back to the midline.
6. Change the orientation of your index finger so that it is now horizontal.
7. While your finger remains in the midline (between the patient's eyes), move your finger smoothly up to assess the patient's vertical upward eye movements.
8. Finally, move your finger smoothly down to assess the patient's vertical downward eye movements.

NORMAL FINDINGS

Normally, each eye should move fully in all of the directions of gaze tested, and both eyes should move together in parallel (i.e., conjugately) in all directions.

ABNORMAL FINDINGS

Findings Due to Disorders of the Cranial Nerves or Extraocular Muscles

Incomplete movement of an eye in the direction of the action of one of the eye muscles suggests dysfunction of that muscle or of the nerve that supplies it. The abnormality can potentially be anywhere within the pathway from the cranial nerve nucleus in the brainstem to the cranial nerve to the neuromuscular junction to the muscle itself. Use the rest of the history and examination (see Chapter 49, Examination of the Patient with Visual Symptoms) to determine where along the pathway the problem most likely arises. There are, however, patterns of findings on the eye movement examination suggestive of particular cranial nerve lesions.

- Incomplete abduction of an eye suggests a lesion of the ipsilateral sixth (abducens) cranial nerve (Fig. 14–1), although dysfunction of the lateral rectus muscle itself could also cause this finding.
- Incomplete adduction, upward movement, and downward movement of an eye suggest a lesion of the ipsilateral third (oculomotor) cranial nerve. When a third nerve palsy is severe, the affected eye deviates laterally and downward (see Fig. 10–1) because of the unopposed actions of the muscles innervated by the sixth and the fourth nerves.
- Oculomotor (third) nerve palsies can be categorized as either *pupillary involving* or *pupillary sparing*, depending on whether the pupillary con-

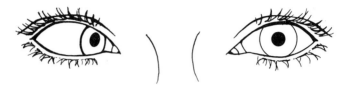

Figure 14-1   Severe weakness of abduction of the left eye in a patient with a left sixth nerve palsy. The patient is trying to follow the examiner's finger to the left.

striction fibers are affected. Oculomotor nerve palsies due to compression of the nerve (such as from an aneurysm or mass lesions) tend to involve the pupil because the pupillary constricting fibers are susceptible as they lie on the outer surface of the nerve; therefore, the pupil may be dilated and unreactive to light (see Fig. 10–1). Oculomotor nerve palsies due to ischemia to the nerve (such as when a patient with diabetes or hypertension has infarction of the nerve due to occlusion of its vascular supply) tend to spare the pupil; therefore, the pupil will likely be symmetric in size compared to the other side and reactive to light.

Abnormalities of Conjugate Gaze

- Severe difficulty for both eyes to look up—upgaze paresis—suggests a lesion of the centers that control vertical gaze in the posterior (dorsal) midbrain/thalamic region, such as from pineal lesions. This finding can be nonspecific, however, especially because diminished upgaze is a common finding in normal aging.
- Severe difficulty for both eyes to look down—downgaze paresis—is an uncommon finding that is primarily associated with the extrapyramidal disorder known as *progressive supranuclear palsy* (see Chapter 46, Examination of the Patient with a Movement Disorder).
- Horizontal gaze palsies—problems with lateral conjugate gaze to one side—are usually associated with the more prominent finding of bilateral sustained deviation of both eyes to the other side (see Chapter 42, Examination of the Comatose Patient).

Other Abnormal Findings

- Nystagmus, a jerking movement of the eyes, is another finding that can be seen while testing eye movements. Nystagmus can be seen in vestibular disorders, such as from peripheral (inner ear) or central (brainstem or cerebellar) vestibulopathies. Nystagmus is described further in Chapter 44, Examination of the Dizzy Patient.
- Incomplete adduction of one eye on attempted lateral gaze (with all other movements of that eye being normal), often accompanied by nystagmus of the abducting eye, is called an *internuclear ophthalmoplegia* (Fig. 14–2). This finding suggests a lesion within the brainstem affecting the medial longitudinal fasciculus, the nerve fiber pathway that connects the sixth cranial nerve on one side of the brainstem to the third cranial nerve on the other side. Internuclear ophthalmoplegias can occur due to any lesion affecting this region of the brainstem, such as from stroke or multiple sclerosis. The finding of a bilateral internuclear ophthalmoplegia, however, is most commonly seen due to multiple sclerosis.

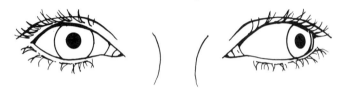

Figure 14-2 Incomplete adduction of the right eye while the patient is trying to look to the left, consistent with a right internuclear ophthalmoplegia. There is also nystagmus of the left (abducting) eye. This patient has a lesion of the right brainstem affecting the right medial longitudinal fasciculus.

ADDITIONAL POINTS

- Complete paralysis of movement of an extraocular muscle is called an *ophthalmoplegia*, and milder weakness of an eye muscle is called an *ophthalmoparesis*.

- It is usually only necessary to look for abnormalities of the medial, lateral, superior, and inferior rectus muscles and to ignore the superior and inferior oblique muscles as you assess eye movements. Trying to assess the action of the oblique muscles adds a level of complexity that is only rarely additionally useful in routine neurologic assessment.

- Because it isn't usually helpful to assess for the action of the oblique muscles, you only need to routinely assess vertical eye movements while the eyes are in the center and not at the extremes of lateral gaze. Check the side-to-side (horizontal) eye movements, then, when the eyes are back in the middle, check the up and down (vertical) eye movements. You don't need to check the corners.

- If you do need to assess the action of the oblique muscles (e.g., if a fourth nerve palsy is suspected clinically), the superior oblique is best tested by having the eye look down while adducted; the inferior oblique is best tested by having the eye look up while adducted. Information about how to recognize the symptoms and signs of a fourth nerve palsy can be found in Chapter 49, Examination of the Patient with Visual Symptoms.

- The eye movements described in this chapter are called *pursuit eye movements*; these are the slow eye movements that are used to track moving objects, like the movements of the examiner's finger. Another type of eye movement, *saccadic eye movement*, is the more rapid movement of the eyes that occurs when quickly changing direction of gaze. In routine neurologic assessment, you only need to assess pursuit eye movements.

Chapter 15

EXAMINATION OF FACIAL SENSATION

PURPOSE

The main purpose of the examination of facial sensation is to assess for lesions involving the fifth (trigeminal) cranial nerve. Another purpose is to assess for lesions of the sensory pathways in the cerebral hemispheres and brainstem that may also cause facial sensory loss.

WHEN TO EXAMINE FACIAL SENSATION

Facial sensation should be tested in any patient who has a symptom of facial numbness or facial pain or in any patient suspected of having a disorder affecting cranial nerves. In patients who have no facial sensory symptoms or when there is no other particular clinical concern for a fifth nerve lesion or a disorder affecting cranial nerves, it is not imperative to test facial sensation routinely.

NEUROANATOMY OF FACIAL SENSATION

Sensation to the face is supplied by the three main branches of the trigeminal nerve: the ophthalmic division (V1, pronounced "vee one"), the maxillary division (V2), and the mandibular division (V3). Figure 15–1 illustrates the cutaneous sensory distributions of the three divisions of the trigeminal nerve.

The trigeminal nerve enters the brainstem at the level of the pons and then synapses with its sensory nucleus; from there, sensory information crosses to the other side to travel to the contralateral thalamus and parietal cortex.

EQUIPMENT NEEDED TO TEST FACIAL SENSATION

- A safety pin and a cotton swab.
- See Chapter 29, Examination of Pinprick Sensation, for details on the use of a safety pin (or appropriate alternative) to test pin sensation.

HOW TO EXAMINE FACIAL SENSATION

1. Test light touch with your finger or with a cotton swab. Simply lightly touch both sides of the patient's forehead (V1) simultaneously and ask if the sensation is "about the same" on each side. Repeat the same question when touching both sides of the patient's cheeks (V2), and when touching both sides of the patient's chin (V3).

2. To test pinprick sensation, inform the patient that you'll be lightly touching the patient's face with the point of the pin, and ask the patient to tell you if the pin sensation is "about the same" on each side. Touch one side of the forehead (V1) with the pin and then the other, and ask the patient if the pin sensation is about the same on each side. Repeat the same process when touching each cheek (V2) and each side of the chin (V3).

NORMAL FINDINGS

Normally, sensation to light touch and pin should be approximately equal on each side of the face, in all three divisions of the trigeminal nerve.

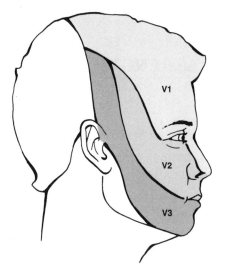

Figure 15–1 The approximate cutaneous sensory distributions of the three divisions of the trigeminal nerve.

ABNORMAL FINDINGS

- Diminished sensation that corresponds to the territory of one or more divisions of the trigeminal nerve on one side of the face suggests a lesion of the trigeminal nerve.
- Diminished sensation of an entire side of the face is suggestive of a central nervous system lesion affecting somatosensory pathways, most likely involving the contralateral thalamus or parietal cortex.

ADDITIONAL POINTS

- The facial sensory examination, as with most sensory tests, is of limited value in the absence of a sensory complaint, such as numbness or tingling. Abnormalities found on facial sensory testing should be interpreted within the clinical context.
- Asking the patient if the sensation to pin or light touch is "about the same" on each side is preferable to asking the patient if there is a "difference" in the sensation on each side. When asked if there is a difference in sensation, the suggestible patient may feel compelled to report (the unavoidable) minor differences in the pressure exerted by the physician, instead of just reporting areas of truly diminished sensation.
- It is a useful general rule that trigeminal neuralgia (paroxysmal pain in the distribution of one or more divisions of the trigeminal nerve) is usually not associated with any significant loss of facial sensation. Actual loss of sensation that maps out one or more divisions of the trigeminal nerve, however, is suggestive of a trigeminal nerve lesion that may be due to significant infiltrative or compressive etiologies.

Chapter 16

EXAMINATION OF FACIAL STRENGTH

PURPOSE

The purpose of the examination of facial strength is to assess for lesions of the central or peripheral nervous system motor pathways that move the face.

WHEN TO EXAMINE FACIAL STRENGTH

All patients should have facial movements assessed as part of a complete neurologic examination. In most patients, the examination of facial symmetry and strength can be limited to observing the patient's smile. For patients who present with a complaint of facial weakness or who show evidence of facial weakness on examination, a more detailed assessment to distinguish upper motor neuron from lower motor neuron weakness should be performed, as described in How to Examine Facial Strength.

NEUROANATOMY OF FACIAL MOVEMENT

The upper motor neuron pathway for facial movement begins in the motor cortex of each frontal lobe. Axons from these nerve cells travel downward as the corticospinal tract, which then synapse at the facial nerve nucleus in the pons. Axons from the facial nucleus—the lower motor neuron for facial movement—leave the pons as the facial nerve to innervate all of the muscles of facial expression on that side of the face. The part of the facial nerve nucleus that moves the lower part of the face (e.g., mouth movement) is innervated mainly by fibers from the contralateral corticospinal tract. The part of the facial nerve nucleus that moves the upper part of the face (e.g., forehead wrinkling and eye closure) is innervated by fibers from both the contralateral and the ipsilateral corticospinal tracts.

EQUIPMENT NEEDED TO TEST FACIAL STRENGTH

None.

HOW TO EXAMINE FACIAL STRENGTH

1. Ask the patient to smile. Assess for any weakness or obvious asymmetry of mouth movement. If no significant facial weakness is seen, the examination of facial strength can end at this step; otherwise, proceed further.
2. Ask the patient to raise his or her eyebrows (show the patient what you mean by wrinkling your own eyebrows). Look for any asymmetry of forehead movement.
3. Ask the patient to close his or her eyes tightly. Look for any obvious asymmetry of strength of eye closure, and assess the ability of the patient to resist your attempt to open his or her eyes.

NORMAL FINDINGS

Normally, there should be full and symmetric movements of the mouth, forehead, and eye closure.

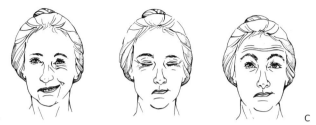

A,B   C

Figure 16–1   A patient with upper motor neuron facial weakness attempting to smile **(A)**, close her eyes **(B)**, and raise her eyebrows **(C)**. The patient has a lesion of the left corticospinal tract causing right-sided facial weakness.

ABNORMAL FINDINGS

- Weakness of the smile on one side of the mouth with normal movement of the forehead muscles and normal eye closure on that side (Fig. 16–1) is consistent with a lesion of the corticospinal tract on the side contralateral to the side of the facial weakness. In other words, a lesion of the left hemisphere (or the left upper brainstem) involving the left corticospinal tract causes weakness of the smile on the right side of the mouth. This is called *upper motor neuron facial weakness.* In upper motor neuron facial weakness, the muscles that move the forehead and close the eye are spared because of the bilateral corticospinal tract innervation to the part of the facial nerve nucleus that performs these functions.
- Weakness of an entire side of the face, including weakness of the smile on one side of the mouth, one side of the forehead, and weakness of closure of the eye (Fig. 16–2), is consistent with a lesion of the facial nerve on that side. In other words, a lesion of the right facial nerve (or its nucleus in the pons) causes right lower motor neuron facial weakness. In lower motor neuron facial weakness, all of the muscles that move the face on one side may be affected because all of these muscles are innervated by the facial nerve on that side.

ADDITIONAL POINTS

- The terminology describing facial weakness can be confusing. Lesions of the upper motor neuron (the corticospinal tract) cause weakness of the

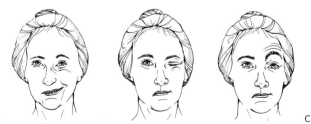

A,B   C

Figure 16–2   A patient with lower motor neuron facial weakness attempting to smile **(A)**, close her eyes **(B)**, and raise her eyebrows **(C)**. The patient has a lesion of the right facial nerve causing right-sided facial weakness.

lower part of the face. Lesions of the lower motor neuron (the facial nerve) cause weakness of the upper and lower parts of the face. Avoid ambiguous terms such as "upper facial" and "lower facial" weakness. It's best to describe facial weakness as upper motor neuron type or lower motor neuron type weakness.

- Patients commonly have a mild asymmetry (often described as *flattening*) of the nasolabial fold on one side of the face compared to the other. The nasolabial fold is the facial crease that extends from the nostril to the corner of the mouth. Mild asymmetry of the nasolabial fold as an isolated finding is usually of doubtful clinical significance.

- The evaluation of taste sensation in patients with possible lower motor neuron facial weakness (such as in Bell's palsy) is described in Chapter 22, Examination of Taste.

- There are some additional unusual findings that may be observed when looking at a patient's resting facial muscles; these should be looked for especially when there is a complaint of abnormal involuntary facial movements.

  - *Hemifacial spasm* consists of intermittent twitches of the muscles on one side of the face, characterized by unilateral eye blinking or twitching of the muscles of one side of the cheek, or both; this generally occurs as a result of compressive dysfunction of a facial nerve.

  - *Facial myokymia* consists of a continuous undulating and quivering movement of the muscles on one side of the face, especially around one eye; this is seen primarily in the setting of multiple sclerosis but has also been described due to brainstem gliomas.

  - *Blepharospasm* consists of intermittent involuntary tight blinking of both eyes; this is a form of focal dystonia (see Chapter 46, Examination of the Patient with a Movement Disorder).

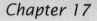

Chapter 17

EXAMINATION OF JAW STRENGTH

PURPOSE

The purpose of the examination of jaw strength is to look for evidence of dysfunction of the motor component of the trigeminal (fifth) nerve in patients who are clinically suspected of having a lesion of this nerve.

WHEN TO EXAMINE JAW STRENGTH

Jaw strength needs to be tested only in patients who are suspected of having trigeminal nerve dysfunction, such as patients who complain of facial numbness.

NEUROANATOMY OF JAW MOVEMENT

The muscles that move the jaw—the masseters and the pterygoids—are supplied by motor branches of the trigeminal (fifth) cranial nerve that originate in the pons and reach the muscles by traveling through the mandibular (V3) division of the nerve. The action of the masseter muscle on each side is to close the jaw. The action of each pterygoid muscle is to pull the jaw forward toward the center; the left pterygoid muscle, therefore, pulls the jaw to the right, and the right pterygoid muscle pulls the jaw to the left.

EQUIPMENT NEEDED TO EXAMINE JAW STRENGTH

None.

HOW TO EXAMINE JAW STRENGTH

1. Ask the patient to open his or her jaw. Note whether the jaw is in the midline or deviates to one side.
2. Next, ask the patient to move the jaw laterally to each side while you try to resist that movement by pushing on the jaw with your hand. Note whether the strength of jaw movement to each side appears approximately the same or is significantly more easily overcome on one side.
3. Ask the patient to close his or her jaw tightly. Palpate both masseter muscles while the patient closes the jaw and assess for symmetry of bulk of these muscles.

NORMAL FINDINGS

- Normally, the jaw should stay in the midline when it opens, and it should not deviate significantly to either side.
- Lateral jaw motion to each side should feel strong and symmetric and not be easily overcome.
- When the patient closes the jaw tightly, the masseter muscles should have symmetric bulk.

ABNORMAL FINDINGS

- Jaw deviation to one side when the mouth is opened is consistent with weakness of the pterygoid muscles on the side that the jaw deviates to. In other words, jaw deviation to the left is consistent with weakness of the left pterygoid muscles and suggests a lesion of the motor fibers of the left trigeminal nerve.
- Weakness of lateral jaw movement to one side suggests weakness of the contralateral pterygoid muscle. In other words, weakness of jaw movement to the left is consistent with right pterygoid muscle weakness and suggests a lesion of the motor fibers of the right trigeminal nerve.
- Diminished bulk of a masseter muscle suggests a lesion involving motor fibers of the ipsilateral trigeminal nerve, causing atrophy of the masseter muscle.

ADDITIONAL POINTS

- Unilateral lesions of the cerebral hemispheres or the brainstem (above the nucleus of the fifth nerve in the pons) do not cause weakness of the muscles that move the jaw because of bilateral upper motor neuron innervation to the fifth nerve nuclei.
- Assessment of motor trigeminal function is of limited value in the routine neurologic examination; in the absence of a specific clinical suspicion of a possible trigeminal nerve lesion, jaw strength does not need to be tested.

Chapter 18

EXAMINATION OF HEARING

PURPOSE

The main purpose of the examination of hearing during the neurologic examination is to assess for gross dysfunction of the acoustic (eighth) nerves.

WHEN TO EXAMINE HEARING

Hearing should be tested when the patient has an auditory complaint or if there is any suspicion of hearing loss. Hearing should also be tested in patients with a possible peripheral vestibular disorder, such as patients with vertigo. In the absence of these scenarios, it is not imperative to test hearing during a routine neurologic examination.

NEUROANATOMY OF HEARING

Sound travels through the external auditory canal to the middle ear and inner ear, where the cochlea converts the sound waves into impulses that travel through the acoustic (eighth) cranial nerve. The eighth nerve reaches the brainstem, where there are extensive bilateral connections with the auditory information from the contralateral eighth nerve. The auditory pathways ascend to reach the auditory cortex in both temporal lobes.

EQUIPMENT NEEDED TO TEST HEARING

A 512-Hz tuning fork.

HOW TO EXAMINE HEARING

Hearing to Finger Rub

1. Have the patient close his or her eyes.
2. Hold your fingers just outside of one ear and rub your fingers gently together so they make a noise. Ask the patient if he or she can hear your fingers rubbing. If the patient cannot hear the sound, increase the intensity of the sound with more vigorous movement of the fingers. Note whether the patient hears gentle finger rubbing in the ear or hears only a louder sound.
3. Repeat the same with the other ear.

Rinne Test to Assess Air Conduction versus Bone Conduction

1. Strike the tuning fork so that the high-pitched sound is audible.
2. Hold the tuning fork just outside of one ear and tell the patient "This is sound number one."
3. Then hold the base of the tuning fork so that it touches the mastoid process of the same ear and tell the patient "This is sound number two."
4. Ask the patient "Which sound was louder? Number one or number two?"
5. Perform the same test on the other ear.

TABLE 18–1 Summary of Examination Findings in Patients with Unilateral Sensorineural or Conductive Hearing Loss in the Left Ear

Cause of Hearing Loss	Hearing (L)	Hearing (R)	Rinne Test (L)	Rinne Test (R)	Weber Test
Sensorineural	Decreased	Normal	AC >BC	AC >BC	Lateralizes to right
Conductive	Decreased	Normal	BC >AC	AC >BC	Lateralizes to left

AC, air conduction; BC, bone conduction; L, left; R, right.

Weber Test to Assess If Sound from a Tuning Fork Lateralizes to One Ear More Than the Other

1. Strike the tuning fork so that you can hear the high-pitched sound fairly loudly.
2. Hold the base of the tuning fork to the center of the patient's forehead.
3. Ask the patient if the sound is heard "pretty much in the center" or if it is heard significantly more in one ear than the other.

NORMAL FINDINGS

Hearing

Normally, the patient should be able to hear your fingers softly rubbing in each ear.

Rinne Test

Normally, the patient should hear the tuning fork louder when it is held outside of the ear than when it is held to the mastoid process. In other words, air conduction (AC) should be better than bone conduction (BC) (AC >BC).

Weber Test

Normally, the patient should hear the sound from the tuning fork in the center of the forehead, approximately equally in both ears, not lateralizing to one ear.

ABNORMAL FINDINGS

Hearing

Difficulty hearing your fingers rubbing is suggestive of hearing loss in that ear, which could be conductive or sensorineural. *Conductive loss* refers to dysfunction of the external ear or the middle ear and its ossicles. *Sensorineural loss* occurs due to dysfunction of the cochlea or the acoustic nerve. Use the findings on Rinne and Weber testing to help you clinically determine whether hearing loss is conductive or sensorineural (as summarized in Table 18–1).

Rinne Test

- The abnormal finding on Rinne testing is that the tuning fork is heard louder when it is held to the mastoid process than when it is held outside the ear [i.e., BC is better than AC (BC >AC)]. This finding on either side is consistent with conductive hearing loss on that side.

- If a patient has hearing loss in an ear, the finding that AC is greater than BC in the ear with hearing loss is consistent with sensorineural (rather than conductive) hearing loss on that side.

Weber Test

- The abnormal finding on Weber testing is that sound lateralizes to one ear. Sound lateralizing to the side with the hearing loss is consistent with conductive hearing loss on that side. In other words, if the left ear has hearing loss, sound lateralizing to the left on Weber testing is consistent with a conductive problem on the left.
- Sound lateralizing away from the side of hearing loss is consistent with sensorineural dysfunction in the ear with hearing loss. In other words, if the left ear has hearing loss, sound lateralizing to the right on Weber testing is consistent with a sensorineural problem on the left.

ADDITIONAL POINTS

- The Rinne test is simple and quick to perform. Many physicians have been trained to perform the test by holding the tuning fork outside the ear until the sound fades and then placing the tuning fork over the mastoid process; this way of performing the test is unnecessarily long. The method described in How to Examine Hearing takes just a few seconds.
- Perform the Weber test on your own ear to see that it really works. Create a "conductive" problem in one ear by holding a finger in one of your ears to block out sound, and then perform the Weber test. You'll find that the sound localizes to the ear that you have occluded.
- Central nervous system lesions rarely cause hearing loss because of the bilateral interconnections of auditory information in the brainstem and cortex.

Chapter 19

EXAMINATION OF PALATAL FUNCTION

PURPOSE

The main purpose of assessment of the palate during the neurologic examination is to look for evidence of dysfunction of the vagus (tenth) nerve. In some cases, palatal movement is assessed to look for evidence of neuromuscular disease causing palatal weakness.

WHEN TO ASSESS PALATAL FUNCTION

Palatal movement should be assessed in most patients as part of a routine neurologic examination. Palatal movement should be particularly assessed in patients who have complaints of difficulty swallowing or slurred speech, or in patients who are suspected of having a severe neuromuscular disorder that may cause palatal weakness. A gag reflex rarely, if ever, needs to be performed on any awake patient as part of a standard neurologic examination, however.

NEUROANATOMY OF PALATAL FUNCTION

Palatal movement occurs because of innervation by the vagus (tenth) nerve of the pharyngeal muscles that elevate the palate. The origin of the vagus nerve is in the medulla. The left vagus nerve innervates the left palatal muscles, and the right vagus nerve innervates the right palatal muscles.

EQUIPMENT NEEDED TO TEST PALATAL FUNCTION

A tongue depressor and a flashlight.

HOW TO EXAMINE PALATAL FUNCTION

1. Ask the patient to open his or her mouth while you look at the patient's soft palate and uvula with a flashlight. If it is difficult to see the palate, gently press down on the tongue with a tongue depressor.
2. Ask the patient to say "ah" (the fancy name for this is *phonation*).
3. Assess the elevation of both sides of the palate and the uvula to phonation.

NORMAL FINDINGS

Normally, both sides of the soft palate should elevate symmetrically when the patient says "ah," and the uvula should remain primarily in the midline.

ABNORMAL FINDINGS

- Limited elevation of one side of the palate occurs due to unilateral palatal weakness and suggests a lesion of the tenth nerve on the weak side. Weakness of elevation of one side of the palate is usually accompanied by deviation of the uvula to the strong side (Fig. 19–1). True unilateral palatal weakness is an uncommon finding, most typically seen in patients with infarctions of the lateral medulla (Wallenberg's syndrome) affecting the nucleus of the tenth cranial nerve or in patients with other disorders

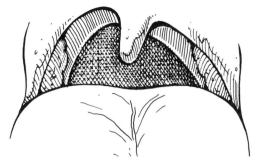

Figure 19-1 Weakness of the left side of the palate in a patient with a left vagus (tenth) nerve lesion. The uvula deviates to the right (strong) side.

affecting the tenth cranial nerve. Vagus nerve lesions causing palatal weakness may also be associated with hoarseness of the voice due to associated unilateral vocal cord weakness.

- Significant weakness of elevation of both sides of the palate can be seen in patients with severe generalized neuromuscular disease, such as myasthenia gravis or Guillain-Barré syndrome. Symptoms of bilateral palatal weakness include a nasal quality to the speech and regurgitation of liquids through the nose when attempting to swallow.
- Palatal myoclonus is a finding that may rarely be seen when looking at the palate and consists of a continuous, rapid, rhythmic jerking of both sides of the soft palate. Palatal myoclonus may be seen due to lesions of the brainstem or as an idiopathic process, and it is sometimes associated with the clinical complaint of a clicking sound in the ears.

ADDITIONAL POINTS

- Patients who have had tonsillectomies may have some asymmetry of their posterior pharynx and soft palate that can sometimes be confused with unilateral palatal weakness. By looking at the palates of many normal patients (including patients with previous tonsillectomies), you'll have a better feel for the normal variations in palatal symmetry.
- Use of the gag reflex in the clinical assessment of brain death is described in Chapter 42, Examination of the Comatose Patient. There is little useful information to be found by testing the gag reflex of a noncomatose patient. The gag reflex is a noxious test and should be avoided in routine neurologic assessment. In those patients in whom swallowing and risk for aspiration needs to be assessed, formal swallowing assessment by a speech therapist should be obtained.

Chapter 20

EXAMINATION OF TONGUE MOVEMENT

PURPOSE

The main purpose of the examination of motor function of the tongue is to look for evidence of dysfunction of the hypoglossal (twelfth) cranial nerve. Another purpose for examination of the tongue is to look for fasciculations, particularly in the clinical context in which motor neuron disease (amyotrophic lateral sclerosis) is a consideration.

WHEN TO EXAMINE TONGUE MOVEMENT

It is appropriate to assess that the tongue protrudes grossly in the midline and that it can wiggle from side-to-side in all patients during a routine neurologic examination. When a patient is being evaluated for the possibility of motor neuron disease, it is also appropriate to specifically inspect the tongue for fasciculations.

NEUROANATOMY OF TONGUE MOVEMENT

The muscles that move the tongue are supplied by the twelfth cranial nerves, which arise from the medial part of the medulla. The left twelfth nerve, which arises from the left medulla, supplies the muscles on the left side of the tongue and moves the tongue to the right. The right twelfth nerve, which arises from the right medulla, supplies the muscles on the right side of the tongue and moves the tongue to the left.

EQUIPMENT NEEDED TO TEST TONGUE MOVEMENT

None (except for a flashlight when needed to look for tongue fasciculations).

HOW TO EXAMINE TONGUE MOVEMENT

1. Ask the patient to stick out his or her tongue.
2. Assess whether the tongue protrudes in the midline or obviously deviates to one side. Look at the tongue for obvious asymmetric atrophy of either side.
3. Ask the patient to wiggle the tongue to one side and then the other.
4. If it appears that there is weakness or unilateral atrophy of the tongue, further assessment of tongue strength can be performed by asking the patient to push the tongue against the inside of one cheek, and then the other, while you assess the resistance of the tongue by pushing against the outside of the cheek with your fingers.
5. To inspect the tongue for fasciculations, ask the patient to relax the tongue on the floor of the mouth, with the tongue resting anteriorly against the lower teeth. Look at the tongue with a flashlight and observe for fasciculations.

NORMAL FINDINGS

Normally, the tongue is approximately midline and does not deviate significantly to either side, moves well to each side, and there is no atrophy or fasciculations.

ABNORMAL FINDINGS

- Obvious deviation of the protruded tongue to one side is consistent with a lesion of a twelfth nerve or its origin in the medulla. Deviation of the tongue to the left would be consistent with a left twelfth nerve lesion, because the "good" right twelfth nerve is unopposed as it pushes the tongue toward the left. Deviation of the tongue to the right would be consistent with a right twelfth nerve lesion.

- Significant asymmetry of ability of the tongue to wiggle to one side or to withstand resistance to the pressure of your finger against the cheek is further evidence for a unilateral twelfth nerve lesion. Weakness of tongue movement toward the left cheek is suggestive of a right twelfth nerve lesion, and weakness of tongue movement toward the right cheek is suggestive of a left twelfth nerve lesion.

- Unilateral twelfth nerve lesions may also be accompanied by atrophy and fasciculations (visible undulating movements of the muscle fibers) of one side of the tongue due to denervation of the intrinsic tongue muscles on that side.

- Bilateral fasciculations of the tongue, usually accompanied by atrophy, may rarely be observed and are typically seen in the setting of motor neuron disease. Tongue fasciculations in this setting are likely to be accompanied by symptoms of slurred speech (dysarthria) and difficulty with swallowing (dysphagia).

ADDITIONAL POINTS

- Lesions of a hypoglossal nerve or the medial medulla are unusual, so it is rare to find significant tongue deviation. Subtle deviation of the tip of the tongue is usually not of clinical significance.

- Lesions within the cerebral hemispheres or upper brainstem don't usually cause significant tongue deviation; this test is, therefore, rarely useful for localization of strokes except in the rare instance when a medullary lesion is suspected.

- Many patients have a subtle tongue tremor that can be mistaken for fasciculations.

Chapter 21

EXAMINATION OF THE STERNOCLEIDOMASTOID AND TRAPEZIUS MUSCLES

PURPOSE

The main purpose of the examination of the sternocleidomastoid and trapezius muscles is to assess for dysfunction of the spinal accessory (eleventh) nerve.

WHEN TO EXAMINE THE STERNOCLEIDOMASTOID AND TRAPEZIUS MUSCLES

Testing of the sternocleidomastoid and trapezius muscles does not need to be performed routinely, but they should be tested in the rare situation when a unilateral lesion of the spinal accessory nerve is suspected. It is also appropriate to test the function of these proximal muscles when assessing for a myopathy or other diffuse neuromuscular process.

NEUROANATOMY OF THE STERNOCLEIDOMASTOID AND TRAPEZIUS MUSCLES

The sternocleidomastoid and trapezius muscles are innervated by the spinal accessory nerve (the spinal portion of the eleventh cranial nerve); this is an unusual cranial nerve because its nuclei originate in the high cervical cord rather than the brainstem. The left sternocleidomastoid muscle turns the head to the right, and the right muscle turns the head to the left; the trapezius muscles shrug the shoulders upward.

EQUIPMENT NEEDED TO TEST THE STERNOCLEIDOMASTOID AND TRAPEZIUS MUSCLES

None.

HOW TO EXAMINE THE STERNOCLEIDOMASTOID AND TRAPEZIUS MUSCLES

1. To test sternocleidomastoid muscle strength, ask the patient to rotate his or her head to one side. Hold your hand on the patient's chin, attempting to overcome the patient's head turn by pushing toward the opposite side. Repeat the same maneuver with the patient turning the opposite direction.
2. To test trapezius muscle strength, ask the patient to shrug his or her shoulders upward. Push down on the patient's shoulders while asking the patient to resist your downward pressure.

NORMAL FINDINGS

Normally, there should be symmetric and strong resistance to your attempt to overcome the patient's sternocleidomastoid and trapezius strength.

ABNORMAL FINDINGS

- Weakness of head turn to one side is consistent with contralateral sterno-cleidomastoid muscle weakness. In other words, weakness of head turn to the left is consistent with weakness of the right sternocleidomastoid muscle due to a lesion of the right eleventh nerve.
- Weakness of shoulder shrug on either side is consistent with ipsilateral trapezius muscle weakness. In other words, weakness of left shoulder shrug is consistent with weakness of the left trapezius muscle due to a lesion of the left eleventh nerve.
- In addition to weakness, atrophy of the sternocleidomastoid or trapezius muscles may be seen when there is a lesion of the eleventh cranial nerve.
- Bilateral weakness of the sternocleidomastoid and trapezius muscles may be seen as a result of proximal muscle weakness from neuromuscular disease.

ADDITIONAL POINTS

- Lesions of the spinal accessory nerve are rare but may occur when the nerve is sectioned iatrogenically (such as during a lymph node resection) or as a result of trauma.
- In the absence of a strong clinical suspicion for a lesion of these nerves or a clinical suspicion for neck and shoulder weakness due to neuromuscular disease, testing the function of these muscles does not add much to the neurologic examination and can usually be skipped.

Chapter 22

EXAMINATION OF TASTE

PURPOSE

The main purpose of testing taste is to look for evidence of dysfunction of the sensory fibers of the facial (seventh) cranial nerve that convey taste from the anterior tongue.

WHEN TO EXAMINE TASTE

Taste needs only to be tested in patients suspected of having peripheral (lower motor neuron) facial weakness or in any patient with a complaint of diminished taste.

NEUROANATOMY OF TASTE

Taste from the anterior two-thirds of the tongue is conveyed by the chorda tympani nerve, which joins the seventh nerve and sends taste sensation to the medulla.

EQUIPMENT NEEDED TO TEST TASTE

Sugar, water, a paper cup, and a tongue depressor (or a cotton swab).

HOW TO EXAMINE TASTE

1. Prepare the sugar mixture outside the patient's view, so that the contents are an unknown. Mix a packet of sugar with a few drops of water so that it has a paste consistency.
2. Explain that you will be testing the patient's ability to taste and that it will not be unpleasant. Ask the patient to close his or her eyes and stick out his or her tongue.
3. Using a tongue depressor or a cotton swab, place some of the paste on one side of the patient's tongue, and ask what he or she tastes. Allow the patient to place the tongue inside the mouth if necessary. Perform the same test on the other side of the tongue. If he or she appropriately detects "sweet" or "sugar" on both sides, also ask the patient if the taste is approximately the same on both sides.

NORMAL FINDINGS

Normally, the patient should be able to taste the sweet sensation on each side of the tongue, and the taste should be approximately equal on both sides.

ABNORMAL FINDINGS

- Diminished or absent taste on one side is abnormal and suggests a lesion of the facial nerve proximal to where the chorda tympani joins it; this finding usually also occurs with other motor signs of a peripheral facial palsy (see Chapter 16, Examination of Facial Strength).
- Absent or significantly diminished taste on both sides of the tongue is an uncommon finding but would be seen in patients with a complaint of diminished taste sensation due to a primary disorder of taste.

ADDITIONAL POINTS

- There is no significant role for testing taste over the posterior tongue, where the taste is carried by the ninth (glossopharyngeal) nerve.
- Not all peripheral facial palsies are associated with diminished taste; however, this finding on the side of a presumed peripheral facial palsy is further evidence for a peripheral origin for the facial weakness, rather than a central origin.

Chapter 23

EXAMINATION OF SMELL

PURPOSE

The purpose of testing smell is to assess for dysfunction of the olfactory (first) cranial nerves.

WHEN TO EXAMINE SMELL

Testing the sense of smell does not need to be performed routinely; in fact, this test rarely needs to be done. Smell should be tested, however, in patients who have a complaint of a diminished sense of smell, in patients in whom a frontal lobe lesion is suspected or known, or in patients with a history of closed head injury or skull fracture.

NEUROANATOMY OF SMELL

Smell receptors in the nasal mucosa send their axons through the cribriform plate to the ipsilateral olfactory bulb, which then sends its axons to the olfactory cortex.

EQUIPMENT NEEDED TO TEST SMELL

Coffee grounds (or other substance with a nonnoxious, recognizable odor).

HOW TO EXAMINE SMELL

1. Put some coffee grounds in a paper cup outside of the patient's view.
2. Ask the patient to close his or her eyes and to cover one nostril. Tell the patient that you will be placing a substance under the open nostril and asking him or her to identify the substance by smell. Inform the patient that it will not be an unpleasant smell.
3. Test the patient's ability to smell the coffee through one nostril and then the other.
4. If the sense of smell is abnormal, confirm that the patient can breathe through each nostril.

NORMAL FINDINGS

Normally, the patient should be able to identify the smell of coffee grounds through each (unobstructed) nostril.

ABNORMAL FINDINGS

- Unilateral absence of smell in the setting of an intact nasal passageway suggests the possibility of ipsilateral olfactory bulb dysfunction, such as can occur as a result of trauma from a basilar skull fracture or compression from an inferior frontal mass.
- Bilateral absence of smell suggests bilateral olfactory nerve dysfunction, which can also be due to traumatic or compressive dysfunction of these nerves but could also be caused by a primary disorder of smell.

ADDITIONAL POINTS

Despite being conveyed by the first cranial nerve, this test is relegated to the last chapter of the cranial nerve section of this book because of how infrequently it needs to be performed. In the appropriate clinical scenarios, however, useful and important information can be learned from this test.

Motor Examination

Chapter 24

APPROACH TO THE MOTOR EXAMINATION

PURPOSE

The purpose of the motor examination is to localize neurologic pathology by looking for characteristic distributions of muscle weakness.

WHEN TO EXAMINE MOTOR FUNCTION

Examination of muscle strength is an essential part of all neurologic examinations and is particularly important in the examination of patients who present with a complaint of weakness. The choice and extent of muscles to be tested should be dictated by the clinical scenario; for example, the muscles that should be examined in a patient in a screening neurologic examination would differ from that of a patient who complains of weakness in an extremity. The assessment for drift of the outstretched arms (see Chapter 25, Examination of Upper Extremity Muscle Strength) should also be performed routinely. Muscle tone, a component of the motor examination that does not need to be assessed in all patients but is helpful in many situations, is described in Chapter 27, Examination of Tone.

NEUROANATOMY OF THE MOTOR EXAMINATION

The pathway for muscle movement begins in nerve cells—the upper motor neurons—located on the precentral gyrus of each frontal lobe. The axons from these nerve cells become the corticospinal tracts, which travel through the internal capsule and into the brainstem; each corticospinal tract then crosses in the low medulla to the opposite side and continues downward through the spinal cord. Within the spinal cord, the corticospinal tracts on each side synapse with nerve cells in the anterior horns of the ipsilateral spinal cord gray matter. Axons from these second-order neurons—the lower motor neurons—leave the spinal cord as the cervical, thoracic, or lumbosacral nerve roots. The nerve roots in the extremities become the brachial or lumbosacral plexus and then the peripheral nerves, which innervate muscles through the neuromuscular junction.

EQUIPMENT NEEDED TO TEST MUSCLE STRENGTH

None.

TABLE 24-1 Grading of Muscle Strength

Grade	Definition
0	Complete paralysis of a muscle
1	Just a trace of muscle movement
2	Muscle movement that cannot overcome the resistance of gravity
3	Muscle can move against gravity but cannot overcome any other resistance
4	Muscle is weak but can move against gravity and additional resistance
5	Normal muscle strength

HOW TO EXAMINE MUSCLE STRENGTH

1. Inspect the muscles for atrophy or fasciculations.
2. Test muscle strength one muscle at a time. It's usually best to test the muscle on one side first and then the other side to assess for symmetry. When weakness on one side is suspected, test the muscle on the strong side before testing the weak side. Sometimes, particularly when focal weakness is not suspected, it's reasonable to test the strength of the same muscles on both sides simultaneously.
3. For each muscle to be tested, ask the patient to hold the limb in the optimal position for testing of that muscle, and instruct the patient to do his or her best to resist as you pull or push in the opposite direction of the action of that muscle, as illustrated and described in Chapter 25, Examination of Upper Extremity Muscle Strength, and Chapter 26, Examination of Lower Extremity Muscle Strength.
4. Grade the strength of each muscle on a scale of 0 (weakest) to 5 (strongest). Table 24-1 summarizes the definition of the grading scale for muscle strength testing.
5. Report the strength of each muscle as its grade out of 5. For example, a muscle with a grade of 4 is reported as 4 out of 5 and is written as 4/5 or, often, simply 4.

NORMAL FINDINGS

Normally, there should be no atrophy or fasciculations of the muscles. Strength should be full (5/5) and symmetric in all muscles tested of the arms and legs.

ABNORMAL FINDINGS

Inspection of the Muscles

Muscle atrophy or fasciculations (visible involuntary twitches of the muscle) are abnormal and suggest dysfunction of the lower motor neuron supplying that muscle; this can occur from a lesion occurring at or anywhere distal to the anterior horn cell, including the motor nerve root, plexus, or peripheral nerve.

Muscle Strength Testing

- Any muscle strength that is less than 5/5 is abnormal. Table 24-2 summarizes the common terminology used to describe muscle weakness.
- Muscle weakness can occur due to upper motor neuron (corticospinal tract) or lower motor neuron dysfunction from lesions located anywhere along the motor pathway from the cerebral cortex to the muscles themselves.

TABLE 24-2 Terminology Used to Describe Muscle Weakness

Terminology	Definition
-*plegia* (suffix)	Paralysis of a muscle or a limb (0/5)
-*paresis* (suffix)	Weakness less severe than complete paralysis (1/5 to 4/5)
Hemiparesis and hemiplegia	Weakness of the arm and leg on one side of the body
Quadriparesis and quadriplegia (sometimes called *tetraplegia*)	Weakness of both arms and both legs
Paraparesis and paraplegia	Weakness of both legs

- Use the distribution of any weakness you discover to help determine the most likely localization of the patient's pathology (Table 24–3).
- As you proceed with the rest of the examination, look for further clues to support or refute your hypothesis regarding the localization of the cause of the patient's weakness, such as the distribution of sensory findings (if any) and the presence or absence of any upper or lower motor neuron signs on reflex testing (see Chapter 36, Approach to Reflex Testing).

ADDITIONAL POINTS

- Although the motor grading scale is easy to understand and use, there's still a significant subjective component to it. There may be significant interphysician and intraphysician variability in muscle grading, even of the same patient.
- Many clinicians like to add a + or a – sign to the muscle grade (for example, 4–) to imply subtle additional distinctions in muscle strength. Be

TABLE 24-3 Lesion Localization Suggested by the Distribution of Weakness

Distribution of Weakness	Localization Suggested
Arm and leg on one side of body (hemiparesis)	Contralateral brain or brainstem
Both arms and both legs (quadriparesis)	Cervical cord (myelopathy), bilateral hemispheres or brainstem, or diffuse neuromuscular process
Both legs (paraparesis)	Spinal cord or cauda equina (or, less likely, both frontal lobes)
Proximal arms and legs	Muscle disease (myopathy) or other diffuse neuromuscular process
Distal arms and legs	Diffuse neuropathic process (polyneuropathy)
Muscles supplied by one nerve root	Nerve root (radiculopathy)
Muscles supplied by portion of brachial or lumbar plexus	Plexus (plexopathy)
Muscles supplied by single peripheral nerve	Single nerve trunk (mononeuropathy)
Muscles supplied by several individual peripheral nerves	Multiple nerve trunks (mononeuropathy multiplex)

aware, however, that many clinicians add the + sign to *all* whole number muscle grades when reporting muscle strength—that is, all muscles with a grade of 4 are written as a 4+. In this situation, only the − sign implies a specific distinction.

- When testing muscle strength, don't be overzealous and wrestle with the patient. It doesn't take a great deal of resistance or power on your part to determine that muscle strength is normal or abnormal or to distinguish a 3 from a 4.

- Save any designation of less than 5 for true muscle weakness and not the giveaway of muscle strength that can occur, for example, due to discomfort or bony or joint pathology. Also, don't grade a patient's normal muscle strength at less than a 5 simply because you are bigger, younger, or stronger than the patient. Most elderly patients, for example, are 5 out of 5 in all muscle groups, unless they have a neurologic problem causing focal or diffuse weakness.

Chapter 25

EXAMINATION OF UPPER EXTREMITY MUSCLE STRENGTH

PURPOSE

The purpose of the examination of upper extremity muscle strength is to localize neurologic pathology by looking for characteristic distributions of muscle weakness.

WHEN TO EXAMINE THE MUSCLE STRENGTH OF THE UPPER EXTREMITIES

A screen of upper extremity strength (see Chapter 40, Performing a Complete Neurologic Examination) should be performed on all patients as part of the routine neurologic examination. If weakness is suspected or found, a more detailed evaluation of upper (and lower) extremity muscles is indicated to try to localize the patient's pathology.

NEUROANATOMY OF THE UPPER EXTREMITY MOTOR EXAMINATION

The upper motor neuron pathways that control the muscles of the upper extremities end primarily within the cervical spinal cord, proceeding no further caudally than the first thoracic level. The lower motor neurons that innervate the muscles of the arms leave the spinal cord primarily from the C5 through the T1 levels. Table 25–1 summarizes the major innervation (root and nerve) of some of the most clinically relevant muscles of the upper extremities, as well as the functions of these muscles.

EQUIPMENT NEEDED TO TEST UPPER EXTREMITY MUSCLE STRENGTH

None.

HOW TO EXAMINE THE MUSCLES OF THE UPPER EXTREMITIES

Test for Drift

Always start the examination of upper extremity strength by testing for drift:
1. Ask the patient to hold his or her arms straight in front of him or her with the palms up.
2. Instruct the patient to close his or her eyes.
3. Observe the arms for a few seconds while the patient's eyes are closed.

Testing Upper Extremity Muscle Strength

Test and grade the muscles of the upper extremities according to the method described in Chapter 24, Approach to the Motor Examination. Figures 25–1 through 25–9 illustrate and describe how to examine some of the major muscle groups of the upper extremities.

TABLE 25-1 Major Innervation of the Muscles of the Upper Extremities

Muscle	Function	Major Root Innervation[a]	Nerve Innervation
Deltoid	Arm abduction	C5	Axillary
Biceps	Elbow flexion	C5, C6	Musculocutaneous
Brachioradialis	Elbow flexion	C6	Radial
Extensor carpi radialis	Wrist extension	C6	Radial
Triceps	Elbow extension	C7	Radial
Extensor digitorum	Finger extension	C7	Radial (posterior interosseus branch)
Flexor pollicis longus	Thumb tip flexion	C8	Median
Flexor digitorum profundus	Second and third fingertip flexion	C8	Median
	Fourth and fifth fingertip flexion	C8	Ulnar
Dorsal interossei	Finger abduction	C8, T1	Ulnar
Abductor pollicis brevis	Thumb abduction	T1	Median

[a]Although muscles share root innervation from several adjacent root levels, this table names the root with the most important, clinically relevant innervation to the given muscle.

NORMAL FINDINGS

Normally, there should be no significant movement (drift) of the outstretched arms when the eyes are closed, and there should be no atrophy or fasciculations of the muscles. Strength should be full (5/5) and symmetric in all muscles tested of the arms.

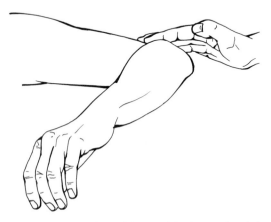

Figure 25-1 Examination of arm abduction (deltoid) strength. Ask the patient to hold his or her arm up 90 degrees at the shoulder ("like a chicken") and then ask the patient to resist you as you push down on his or her abducted arm. What you might say as you test the strength: "Don't let me push your arm down."

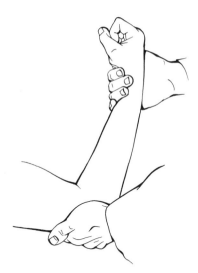

Figure 25-2 Examination of elbow flexion (biceps) strength. Ask the patient to flex his or her arm at approximately 90 degrees at the elbow, with his or her palm facing the shoulder ("like you are making a muscle"), and then ask the patient to resist you as you attempt to extend his or her arm. What you might say as you test the strength: "Don't let me pull on your arm."

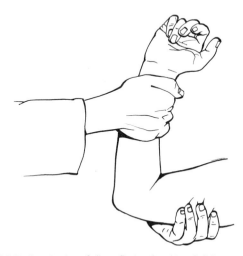

Figure 25-3 Examination of elbow flexion (brachioradialis) strength. Ask the patient to flex his or her arm at approximately 90 degrees at the elbow, with the patient's forearm partially pronated so that the radial wrist is facing his or her shoulder, and then ask the patient to resist you as you attempt to extend the arm. What you might say as you test the strength: "Don't let me pull on your arm."

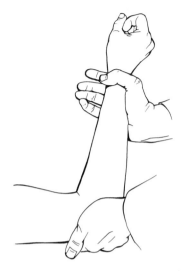

Figure 25–4 Examination of elbow extension (triceps) strength. Ask the patient to start with his or her arm bent at approximately 90 degrees at the elbow, and then as you push on his or her arm, ask the patient to try to push the arm out (by extending at the elbow) against your resistance. What you might say as you test the strength: "Try to push your arm out."

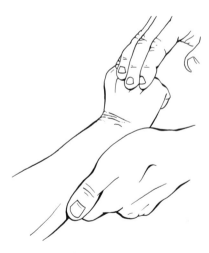

Figure 25–5 Examination of wrist extension (extensor carpi radialis and extensor carpi ulnaris) strength. Ask the patient to lift (extend) his or her hand at the wrist, and then ask the patient to resist you as you attempt to push down on his or her extended hand. What you might say as you test the strength: "Don't let me push your hand down."

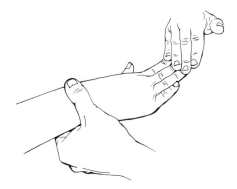

Figure 25–6 Examination of finger extension (extensor digitorum communis) strength. Ask the patient to lift (extend) his or her fingers, and then ask the patient to resist you as you attempt to push down on the extended fingers. What you might say as you test the strength: "Don't let me push your fingers down."

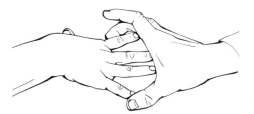

Figure 25–7 Examination of finger abduction (dorsal interossei) strength. Ask the patient to spread his or her fingers apart, and then ask the patient to resist you as you use your thumb and middle finger to attempt to close his or her fingers. What you might say as you test the strength: "Don't let me squeeze your fingers together."

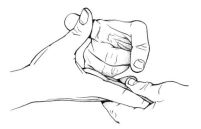

Figure 25–8 Examination of thumb abduction (abductor pollicis brevis) strength. Ask the patient to lift his or her thumb up (perpendicular to the plane of the palm), and then ask the patient to resist as you attempt to push the thumb down. What you might say as you test the strength: "Don't let me push your thumb down."

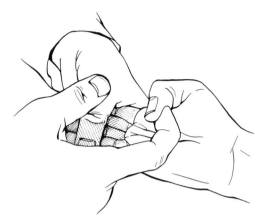

Figure 25–9 Examination of thumb flexion (flexor pollicis longus) strength. Ask the patient to flex the distal joint of the thumb, and then ask the patient to resist you as you attempt to straighten the thumb. (Similar testing can be done to test the flexor digitorum profundus that flexes the distal phalanx of the fingers.) What you might say as you test the strength: "Don't let me pull your thumb."

ABNORMAL FINDINGS

Testing for Drift

- The finding of any downward drift of an arm when the patient's eyes are closed suggests weakness of that extremity due to any cause.
- Downward drift of an arm can occur with or without pronation. When it occurs with pronation, the term *pronator drift* is often used. Whether the downward drift occurs with or without pronation, the significance—weakness—is the same.
- Rarely, when drift is tested, an arm may assume unusual posturing at multiple joints, sometimes with significant upward movement. This finding suggests the possibility of a proprioceptive problem (see Chapter 30, Examination of Vibration and Position Sensation), as can be seen from disorders of the spinal cord, sensory nerves or roots, or contralateral parietal lobe.

Strength

- Any muscle strength in the arms that is less than 5/5 is abnormal.
- Any focal muscle atrophy or fasciculations in the muscles of the arms is abnormal and suggests dysfunction of the lower motor neuron supplying those muscles.
- Look for patterns of muscle weakness (in the arms as well as the legs) to support or refute your suspicion of the localization of the cause of weakness to the brain, spinal cord, root, plexus, or nerve (see Table 24–3).

ADDITIONAL POINTS

- The test for drift is an important part of the motor examination because even subtle downward drift of an arm suggests weakness in that extremity, even before you perform any individual muscle strength testing. Think of drift as the sneak preview to the motor examination. Finding drift suggests there is subtle extremity weakness regardless of whether further evidence for weakness is seen on muscle testing.

- The muscles described in this chapter are not inclusive of all the muscles of the arms that may need to occasionally be tested to localize a cause of weakness, but they do represent muscles that are particularly helpful to have a working knowledge of for the majority of neurologic examinations.

Chapter 26

EXAMINATION OF LOWER EXTREMITY MUSCLE STRENGTH

PURPOSE

The purpose of the examination of lower extremity muscle strength is to localize neurologic pathology by looking for characteristic distributions of muscle weakness.

WHEN TO EXAMINE THE MUSCLE STRENGTH OF THE LOWER EXTREMITIES

A screen of lower extremity strength (see Chapter 40, Performing a Complete Neurologic Examination) should be performed on all patients as part of the routine neurologic examination. If weakness is suspected or found, a more detailed evaluation of lower (and upper) extremity muscles is indicated to try to localize the patient's pathology.

NEUROANATOMY OF THE LOWER EXTREMITY MOTOR EXAMINATION

The upper motor neuron pathways that control the muscles of the lower extremities end primarily within the lumbar spinal cord, proceeding no further caudally than the first sacral level. The lower motor neurons that innervate the muscles of the legs leave the spinal cord primarily from the L1 through S1 levels. Table 26–1 summarizes the major innervation (root and nerve) of some of the most clinically relevant muscles of the lower extremities, as well as the functions of these muscles.

EQUIPMENT NEEDED TO TEST LOWER EXTREMITY MUSCLE STRENGTH

None.

HOW TO EXAMINE THE MUSCLES OF THE LOWER EXTREMITIES

Test and grade the muscles of the lower extremities according to the method described in Chapter 24, Approach to the Motor Examination. Figures 26–1 through 26–9 illustrate and describe how to examine some of the major muscle groups of the lower extremities.

NORMAL FINDINGS

Normally, there should be no atrophy or fasciculations of the muscles, and strength should be full (5/5) and symmetric in all muscles tested of the lower extremities.

ABNORMAL FINDINGS

Strength

- Any muscle strength in the legs that is less than 5/5 is abnormal.

TABLE 26–1 Major Innervation of the Muscles of the Lower Extremities

Muscle	Function	Major Root Innervation[a]	Nerve Innervation
Iliopsoas	Hip flexion	L1, L2, L3	Femoral
Quadriceps	Knee extension	L2, L3, L4	Femoral
Adductors	Hip adduction	L2, L3, L4	Obturator
Hamstrings	Knee flexion	L5, S1	Sciatic
Tibialis anterior	Foot dorsiflexion	L4, L5	Peroneal
Tibialis posterior	Foot inversion	L4, L5	Tibial
Extensor hallucis longus	Large toe dorsiflexion	L5	Peroneal
Peroneus longus	Foot eversion	L5, S1	Peroneal
Gastrocnemius	Foot plantar flexion	S1, S2	Tibial

[a]This table names the roots with the most important, clinically relevant innervation to the given muscle.

- Any focal muscle atrophy or fasciculations in the muscles of the legs is abnormal and suggests dysfunction of the lower motor neuron supplying those muscles.
- Look for patterns of muscle weakness (in the legs as well as the arms) to support or refute your suspicion of the localization of the cause of weakness to the brain, spinal cord, root, plexus, or nerve (see Table 24–3).

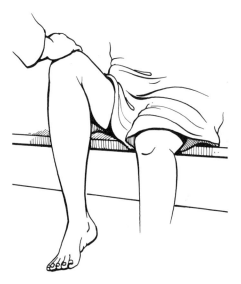

Figure 26–1 Examination of hip flexor (iliopsoas) strength. Ask the patient to lift his or her thigh off of the bed or examining table, and then ask the patient to resist you as you try to push the thigh down. What you might say as you test the strength: "Don't let me push your thigh down."

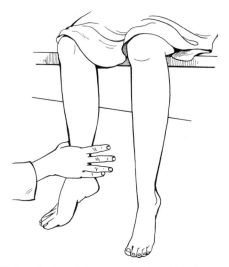

Figure 26–2 Examination of knee extensor (quadriceps) strength. Starting with the patient's leg bent (flexed) at the knee, ask him or her to attempt to extend the leg at the knee against your resistance. What you might say as you test the strength: "Push your leg against me."

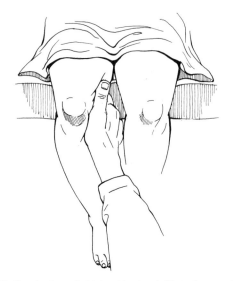

Figure 26–3 Examination of thigh adduction (adductor) strength. Starting with the patient's thigh relatively parallel to the trunk, ask the patient to resist you as you attempt to abduct his or her thigh. What you might say as you test the strength: "Keep your thigh in the center, and don't let me pull it to the side."

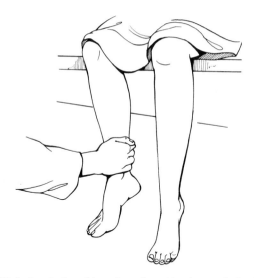

Figure 26–4 Examination of knee flexor (hamstrings) strength. Starting with the patient's leg bent (flexed) at the knee, ask him or her to resist your attempt to straighten the leg. What you might say as you test the strength: "Don't let me straighten your leg."

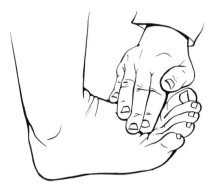

Figure 26–5 Examination of foot dorsiflexor (tibialis anterior) strength. Ask the patient to lift his or her foot up by bending at the ankle, and then ask him or her to resist you as you attempt to push down on the foot. What you might say as you test the strength: "Don't let me push your foot down."

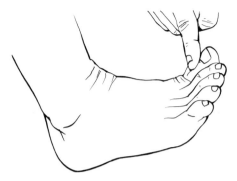

Figure 26–6 Examination of large toe dorsiflexor (extensor hallucis longus) strength. Ask the patient to lift his or her large toe upward, and then ask him or her to resist you as you attempt to push the toe down. What you might say as you test the strength: "Don't let me push your toe down."

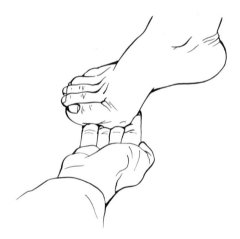

Figure 26–7 Examination of foot plantar flexion (gastrocnemius) strength. Ask the patient to push his or her foot down, bending at the ankle ("as if you are pushing on a gas pedal") and then ask the patient to resist you as you push upward on the sole. What you might say as you test the strength: "Don't let me push your foot up."

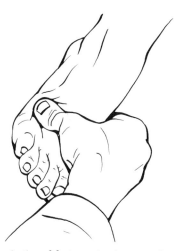

Figure 26–8 Examination of foot eversion (peroneus longus) strength. Ask the patient to turn his or her foot outward and upward at the ankle, lifting the lateral foot upward, and then ask the patient to resist you as you attempt to push downward on the lateral foot. What you might say as you test the strength: "Don't let me push down on your foot."

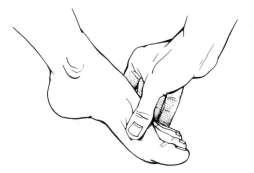

Figure 26–9 Examination of foot inversion (tibialis posterior) strength. Ask the patient to turn his or her foot inward at the ankle, lifting the medial foot upward, and then ask the patient to resist you as you attempt to push downward on the medial foot. What you might say as you test the strength: "Don't let me push down on your foot."

ADDITIONAL POINTS

The muscles described in this chapter are not inclusive of all the muscles of the legs that may need to occasionally be tested to localize a cause of weakness, but they do represent muscles that are particularly helpful to have a working knowledge of for the majority of neurologic examinations.

Chapter 27

EXAMINATION OF TONE

PURPOSE

The purpose of the examination of tone is to assess for spasticity that can occur due to disorders of the corticospinal tract or for rigidity that can be seen in parkinsonism.

WHEN TO EXAMINE TONE

Tone does not need to be assessed routinely; however, muscle tone should be examined in patients who complain of weakness or stiffness in the extremities, in patients with abnormalities of gait, or in patients in whom a basal ganglia disorder is suspected.

NEUROANATOMY OF MUSCLE TONE

Spasticity

When a patient's limb is passively flexed or extended at a joint, muscle spindles and Golgi tendon organs respond to the change in muscle length and initiate a reflex that sends impulses to agonist or antagonist muscles to maintain the appropriate resistance to movement. The corticospinal tract has an inhibitory influence on this spinal reflex mechanism; therefore, upper motor neuron lesions may cause an increase in tone in the affected limbs called *spasticity*.

Rigidity

Whereas lesions of the corticospinal tract (pyramidal dysfunction) can cause spasticity, lesions of the basal ganglia (extrapyramidal dysfunction) can cause an increase in tone called *rigidity*. Rigidity due to extrapyramidal dysfunction is usually described as *cogwheeling*, which is detailed in Abnormal Findings.

EQUIPMENT NEEDED TO ASSESS MUSCLE TONE

None.

HOW TO EXAMINE TONE

Test for Spasticity

1. The test for spasticity is generally performed in the lower extremities. Have the patient lie supine in bed or on an examining table, with legs extended.
2. Test one leg at a time. Place your hands underneath your patient's thigh and lift the patient's thigh up quickly in an attempt to cause flexion of the leg at the knee. Observe the response of the patient's lower leg to this maneuver.
3. Perform the same maneuver on the other leg.
4. With the patient still supine, additional testing for spasticity can include passively flexing the patient's knee joint, feeling for resistance to this maneuver. The same test can be done in the upper extremities by attempting to passively extend the patient's elbow.

Test for Rigidity

1. Rigidity is generally tested in the upper extremities, with the patient sitting or standing.
2. Test one arm at a time. To test the patient's left arm, rest the patient's elbow in your left hand, with your left thumb touching the patient's biceps tendon. Grasp the patient's wrist with your right hand.
3. Move the patient's arm by gently flexing and extending (including some rotational motion as well) the patient's arm at the elbow and the wrist. Note the tone at the elbow and the wrist as you perform this maneuver.
4. Repeat the same procedure (using your opposite hands) on the patient's other arm.

NORMAL FINDINGS

Examination for Spasticity

Normally, if the patient is relaxed, his or her heel should fall to the examining table when the thigh is lifted. There should also be no significant involuntary resistance when you passively flex the patient's knee or extend the patient's arm at the elbow.

Examination for Rigidity

Normally, you should not feel any significant involuntary resistance to passive flexion, extension, or rotational motion of the patient's wrist or elbow.

ABNORMAL FINDINGS

Examination for Spasticity

- Increased tone from spasticity at the knee joint is suggested if the foot stays up (i.e., the knee joint stays extended) when you lift the patient's thigh, hesitating at least briefly before falling to the bed. This finding is called a *spastic catch*.
- Spasticity also may manifest as *clasp-knife* rigidity when you attempt to passively flex the patient's knee (or extend at the elbow). Clasp-knife rigidity consists of initially strong muscle resistance followed by a sudden loss of that resistance.
- The finding of spasticity suggests dysfunction of the corticospinal tract anywhere from its origin in the brain through its descent in the spinal cord. Spasticity in the lower extremities predominantly involves leg extensors, and spasticity in the upper extremities predominantly involves arm flexors.

Examination for Rigidity

- *Cogwheel rigidity* is a ratchety resistance to your passive movement of the patient's wrist or elbow and suggests a basal ganglia disorder, such as Parkinson's disease (see Chapter 46, Examination of the Patient with a Movement Disorder). In addition to cogwheeling, patients with extrapyramidal dysfunction can have a general increase in tone in the extremities.
- Another kind of rigidity that can sometimes be seen is *gegenhalten*, in which the harder you try to flex or extend the patient's elbow, the greater the resistance you feel. This is analogous to variable resistance exercise equipment, which provides greater resistance as one increases the force applied. Gegenhalten rigidity can be seen in severe dementias and is considered a sign of frontal lobe dysfunction.

ADDITIONAL POINTS

- Spasticity is usually accompanied by other signs of upper motor neuron dysfunction, such as weakness, hyperreflexia, and Babinski signs (see Chapters 36 through 38). The finding of spasticity usually implies some chronicity, as it may take days to weeks for spasticity to develop after an upper motor neuron lesion.
- Rigidity due to basal ganglia disorders is usually accompanied by other signs of extrapyramidal dysfunction, such as a parkinsonian gait or tremor (see Chapter 46, Examination of the Patient with a Movement Disorder).
- Although this chapter focuses on assessing tone to find hypertonia, *hypotonia* (a marked reduction of muscle tone) can also be seen. Hypotonia can occur due to severe lower motor neuron or sensory dysfunction affecting the muscle stretch reflex arc, so it can be seen mainly in the setting of severe peripheral motor or sensory nerve lesions.

Sensory Examination

Chapter 28

APPROACH TO THE SENSORY EXAMINATION

PURPOSE

The main purpose of the sensory examination is to localize neurologic pathology by looking for characteristic distributions of sensory loss.

WHEN TO PERFORM THE SENSORY EXAMINATION

A detailed sensory examination, including testing for pin and vibratory sensation, should be performed on any patient who presents with sensory symptoms, such as numbness or tingling in a part of the body or extremities. A detailed sensory examination should also be performed on any patient with signs or symptoms of any focal disorder of the central of peripheral nervous system, because the finding of associated sensory loss may aid in localization.

In patients without sensory symptoms or other significant focal neurologic symptoms or signs, however, the sensory examination plays a limited role. In these patients, an assessment of distal vibratory sensation usually suffices to confirm normal sensory function.

NEUROANATOMY OF SENSATION

The sensory pathways for the body and the extremities begin in peripheral receptors, travel up the peripheral nerves to the dorsal nerve roots, and then enter the spinal cord. In the spinal cord, the sensory pathways ascend as the *spinothalamic tract* (mainly subserving pain and temperature sensation; see Chapter 29, Examination of Pinprick Sensation) and the *posterior columns* (mainly subserving vibration and proprioceptive sensation; see Chapter 30, Examination of Vibration and Position Sensation). After ascending in the spinal cord, these tracts synapse in the contralateral thalamus, where the sensory information is then relayed to the cerebral cortex.

Dermatomes are the areas of skin where the sensation is supplied by a single nerve root. Dermatome charts (Fig. 28–1) summarize the approximate cutaneous sensory territory of nerve root innervation of the body and the extremities. These charts are helpful in localizing patients' sensory symptoms to the appropriate region when those symptoms are due to a lesion of the nerve root or the spinal cord. The cutaneous distribution of the peripheral nerves themselves (Fig. 28–2) can also be shown graphically and can aid in localization of patients' sensory symptoms to a particular peripheral nerve lesion.

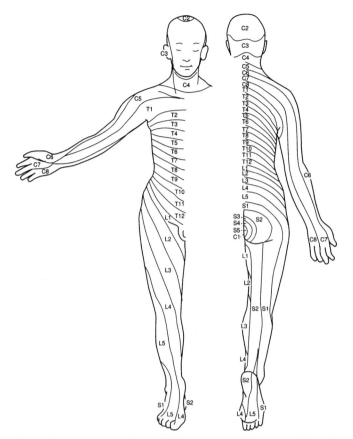

Figure 28-1 Dermatome chart of the anterior and posterior body and extremities. (From Dudek RW. *High-yield gross anatomy.* Philadelphia: Williams & Wilkins, 1997.)

EQUIPMENT NEEDED TO TEST SENSATION

- 256-Hz tuning fork
- Safety pin (see Chapter 29, Examination of Pinprick Sensation, for details on the use of a safety pin or appropriate alternative to test pin sensation)

HOW TO EXAMINE SENSATION

The specifics of how to examine sensation to pin, vibration, and proprioception are discussed in Chapter 29, Examination of Pinprick Sensation, and Chapter 30, Examination of Vibration and Position Sensation. In general, though, the approach to performing the sensory examination should vary depending on the clinical suspicion of lesion localization as your thought process evolves during the history and examination.

- If you suspect a brain, thalamic, or brainstem localization, concentrate on detecting side-to-side differences in sensation.
- If you suspect a spinal cord localization of the patient's symptoms, concentrate on detecting a decrease in sensation below a dermatomal level (see Chapter 51, Examination of the Patient with a Suspected Spinal Cord Problem).
- If you suspect a nerve root localization of symptoms, concentrate on assessing sensation within the dermatome of the nerve root of concern, comparing it to other nerve root distributions on the same side and on the other side.
- If you suspect a lesion of a specific nerve, concentrate on assessing sensation within the distribution of that nerve, comparing it to the sensation within areas supplied by other nerves on the same side and the other side.
- If you suspect a polyneuropathy, concentrate on assessing the extremities for a change in sensation distally compared to proximally.

NORMAL FINDINGS

Normally, patients should feel all sensory modalities equally on both sides of the body, within all cutaneous distributions, and sensation should be the same distally, as well as proximally.

ABNORMAL FINDINGS

- Any alteration in sensation is potentially abnormal. Abnormal findings on sensory testing may include loss of sensation or an abnormally painful sensation to the sensory stimulus being tested. Table 28–1 summarizes some of the terminology used to describe sensory findings.
- Use the distribution of any sensory abnormality you discover (and the distribution of the patient's subjective sensory symptoms) to help you determine the most likely localization of your patient's pathology. Table 28–2 summarizes the localizations suggested by different distributions of sensory signs and symptoms.
- Use the rest of the neurologic examination (particularly the motor and reflex components) to look for further evidence to support or refute your hypothesis obtained from sensory testing regarding the localization of pathology.

ADDITIONAL POINTS

- The sensory examination is of limited value in the absence of a sensory complaint, such as numbness or tingling, or in the absence of a suspicion of a process that may cause sensory findings. Abnormalities found on the sensory examination should be interpreted within the clinical context.
- When comparing sensation in one area to another, it is preferable to ask the patient if the sensation is "about the same" in each area rather than asking the patient if there is a "difference" in the sensation. When asked if there is a difference in sensation, the suggestible patient may feel compelled to report inadvertent minor differences in the pressure exerted by the physician, instead of just reporting areas of truly diminished sensation.

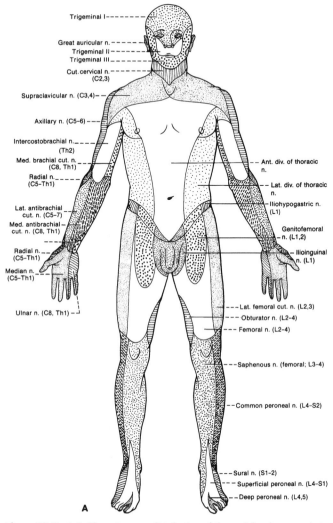

Figure 28–2 A,B: The cutaneous distribution of the peripheral nerves. Ant., anterior; C, cervical; cut., cutaneous; div., division; L, lumbar; lat., lateral; med., medial; n., nerve; post., posterior; S, sacral; Th, thoracic. *Continued.*

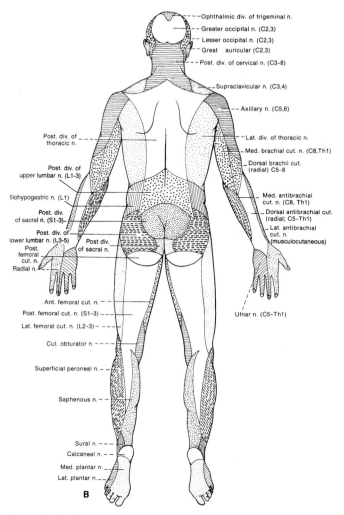

Figure 28-2 *Continued.* (From Haerer A. *DeJong's the neurologic examination.* Philadelphia: JB Lippincott Co, 1992:56–57.)

TABLE 28–1 Terminology Used to Describe Sensory Examination Findings

Finding	Terminology
Absent sensation	Anesthesia
Diminished sensation	Hypesthesia
Increased sensation	Hyperesthesia
Painful sensation	Dysesthesia

TABLE 28–2 Lesion Localization by Distribution of Sensory Examination Findings and Sensory Symptoms

Distribution of Sensory Signs or Symptoms	Localization Suggested
One side of the body (hemisensory loss)	Contralateral brain or thalamus
One side of the body and the other side of the face	Brainstem (ipsilateral to the loss of facial sensation)
Both sides of body below a dermatomal level (sensory level)	Spinal cord
Distribution of a single nerve root	Nerve root
Distribution of a single peripheral nerve	Single peripheral nerve
Distal extremities	Polyneuropathy

Chapter 29

EXAMINATION OF PINPRICK SENSATION

PURPOSE

The main purpose of the examination of pinprick sensation is to localize neurologic pathology by looking for characteristic distributions of pinprick loss.

WHEN TO EXAMINE PINPRICK SENSATION

Examination of pinprick sensation should be performed on any patient who has a sensory complaint, such as numbness or tingling. Pinprick testing should also be performed on most patients with signs or symptoms of any focal disorder of the central or peripheral nervous system, because the finding of associated pin loss may aid in localization. Examination of pinprick sensation otherwise does not need to be performed routinely in all patients.

NEUROANATOMY OF PIN SENSATION

The pathway for pinprick sensation begins in sensory nerve endings in the skin, travels up the peripheral nerves to the dorsal nerve roots to enter the spinal cord and, immediately after entering, crosses to the other side of the cord and becomes the *spinothalamic tract*. The spinothalamic tract ascends the spinal cord and synapses in the thalamus, where the sensory information for pin sensation is relayed to the parietal cerebral cortex. In other words, pin sensation felt on the left side of the body ascends the right side of the spinal cord and ends up in the right thalamus and right sensory cortex.

EQUIPMENT NEEDED TO TEST PIN SENSATION

- A safety pin (preferred) or the point of a broken wooden cotton swab.
- Make sure that the pin is fresh from the factory and has not been used before. It is mandatory that the pin (or pointed stick) be used only on your one patient, and it should be discarded in a sharps container after use. Never use a hypodermic needle to test pin sensation (these are too sharp and draw blood), and never use any nondisposable pins, such as pins that come screwed into the top of some reflex hammers.

HOW TO EXAMINE PINPRICK SENSATION

1. Inform the patient that you'll be lightly touching his or her skin with the point of a pin and that it shouldn't hurt (because it shouldn't hurt if you test for pin sensation correctly). Tell the patient that you will be asking if the pin sensation feels about the same in terms of "pointedness" in different areas compared to others. The patient's eyes can remain open when assessing pinprick sensation with the method described here.
2. Lightly touch the area of skin you want to test with the point of the pin, asking the patient if he or she feels the "pointedness" of the pin. Never scratch the skin or press hard enough that it would be truly noxious or draw blood. When comparing one area of skin to another, ask if the "pointedness is about the same" or not. If the patient reports a difference in sensation, ask the patient to describe the difference to you.

3. Plan your examination of pin sensation depending on your diagnostic suspicion, based on your patient's symptoms and the preceding and evolving examination findings.

   • If you suspect a possible brain, thalamic, or brainstem localization of your patient's symptoms, concentrate on detecting side-to-side differences in pin sensation. To do this, test pinprick sensation once on one arm, then ask the patient if the pin feels about the same as you test the same area of the opposite arm to a single pinprick. This can be tested in a few areas of one arm (or body) and compared to the other side, checking the sensation to an area on one side first and then checking its mirror image. Do the same in the lower extremities by testing pin sensation on one leg compared to the other.

   • If you suspect a spinal cord localization of your patient's symptoms, concentrate on detecting a decrease in sensation below a dermatomal level. For example, if you think there is a possible thoracic cord localization, march the pin down one side of the chest and abdomen by testing single pinpricks scattered inches apart while asking the patient if the pointedness feels about the same as you go down. Do the same on each side of the chest and abdomen, anteriorly and posteriorly.

   • If you suspect a nerve root localization, concentrate on checking pin sensation within the dermatome of the nerve root of concern (depending on the patient's symptoms), comparing to other nerve root distributions. To do this, check the patient's sensation to pinprick within several areas of the extremity (or body) that likely belong to the involved dermatome (see Fig. 28–1), then ask the patient if the pinprick sensation is about the same or different as you assess pinprick in other dermatomes in the same extremity and the opposite extremity.

   • If you suspect a lesion of a specific nerve, concentrate on assessing sensation to pinprick within the distribution of that nerve (see Fig. 28–2), comparing it to the sensation to pin within areas supplied by other nerves of the same extremity and the other extremity, analogous to the assessment of nerve root sensory loss.

   • If you suspect a polyneuropathy, concentrate on checking for a change in sensation in the distal extremities compared to the proximal extremities. Because most polyneuropathies are worse in the lower extremities, test for distal sensory loss by marching the pin down one leg, starting in the calf or thigh and proceeding down to the toes. Test with single pinpricks spaced a few inches apart as you go down. Make sure that the patient can define the pin as "sharp" or "pointed" wherever you start proximally, then ask if the pinprick is about the same or less sharp as you proceed distally. Do the same test on the other leg.

4. It is often helpful to assist patients in their description of a sensory change to pinprick. Patients usually have little difficulty reporting that the sensation is decreased or otherwise altered (e.g., tingly or uncomfortable). When they report that the sensation is decreased, however, you may want to quantify this to help you determine how clinically significant the decrease is. One way to do this is to touch the patient with the pin in an area that the patient has reported as being normal and tell the patient "This is 100% of pointedness." Then, touch the patient with the pin in an area that the patient has reported as having a decrease in sensation and ask "What percent of pointedness is this?"

NORMAL FINDINGS

Normally, patients should feel pinprick equally on both sides of the body, within all cutaneous distributions, and sensation should be the same distally as proximally.

ABNORMAL FINDINGS

- A difference in sensation to pinprick in one area of the body compared to another is abnormal. This difference could be a feeling of diminished sensation (hypesthesia or anesthesia) or other altered sensation (hyperesthesia or dysesthesia). Areas of diminished sensation are more likely to be of clinical significance the greater the patient's subjective quantification of that decrease (i.e., a hypesthetic area described as 50% of normal is more likely to be a significant finding than one described as 90% of normal).

- A difference in pinprick sensation of the extremities or body on one side compared to the other side suggests a brain, thalamic, or brainstem localization of symptoms. The side of the body that shows the diminished or altered sensation is the abnormal side and would be contralateral to the central nervous system lesion. (Hemi-spinal cord lesions would also cause a unilateral decrease in pinprick sensation on one side of the body contralateral to the lesion, but there would also be a loss of posterior column sensation on one side of the body ipsilateral to the lesion; see Chapter 51, Examination of the Patient with a Suspected Spinal Cord Problem.)

- A decrease or other altered sensation to pinprick below a dermatomal level suggests a spinal cord localization of symptoms. The dermatomal level where the sensory loss begins to change represents the patient's *sensory level.* The sensory level found on examination represents the lowest possible level of the patient's spinal cord lesion (the actual level of the lesion might be somewhere above the dermatomal level found; see Chapter 51, Examination of the Patient with a Suspected Spinal Cord Problem).

- A decrease or other altered sensation to pinprick confined to the distribution of a nerve root suggests a nerve root (radicular) lesion at that level.

- A decrease or other altered sensation to pinprick confined to the distribution of an individual peripheral nerve suggests a lesion of that nerve.

- A decrease or other altered sensation to pinprick confined to the distal aspects of the extremities suggests a polyneuropathy. If the distal sensory change is only found in the legs, this is called a *stocking pattern of sensory loss*; when more severe, the sensory change may also be found in the distal upper extremities and is called a *stocking-glove pattern.*

ADDITIONAL POINTS

- Another method of pinprick testing involves asking the patient to discriminate "sharp" from "dull" by asking the patient to close his or her eyes, then asking the patient if you are touching the skin with the sharp side (point) of the pin or the dull side (the side of the safety pin opposite the point). This method is more time-consuming, and differences between areas can't as easily be compared; however, this way to assess pin sensation can be useful as an adjunct to confirm any sensory loss suggested by the method described in How to Examine Pinprick Sensation.

- Another important modality mediated by the same pathways as pinprick sensation is the perception of temperature sensation. Temperature sensation rarely needs to be assessed, but testing for this modality is helpful in the clinical assessment of spinal cord lesions, particularly hemi-spinal cord lesions (the Brown-Séquard syndrome), discussed in Chapter 51, Examination of the Patient with a Suspected Spinal Cord Problem.

Chapter 30

EXAMINATION OF VIBRATION AND POSITION SENSATION

PURPOSE

The main purpose of the examination of vibration and position (proprioception) sense is to assess for evidence of dysfunction of the peripheral sensory nerves in the extremities or the sensory pathways in the spinal cord.

WHEN TO EXAMINE VIBRATION AND POSITION SENSATION

Testing of vibratory sensation should be performed in all patients as part of a routine neurologic examination. Testing of vibration sense is particularly important in patients with sensory symptoms, such as numbness or tingling, or in any patient being assessed for the possibility of a peripheral nerve or spinal cord process.

Testing for position sense probably does not need to be performed routinely; however, position sense should be tested in all patients who have sensory symptoms, in patients who have significant sensory findings to vibration or pin, or in patients with a complaint of problems with gait or balance.

NEUROANATOMY OF VIBRATION AND POSITION SENSE

The pathways for vibration and joint position sense begin in peripheral sensory receptors. Information from these receptors travels up the peripheral nerves to the dorsal roots to enter the spinal cord, ascends the ipsilateral spinal cord as the posterior columns, crosses to the contralateral side in the low medulla, and then ascends through the brainstem to reach the thalamus and the parietal cortex. In other words, vibration and proprioceptive sensation felt on the left side ascends the left posterior spinal cord and crosses in the medulla to end up in the right thalamus and right sensory cortex.

EQUIPMENT NEEDED TO TEST VIBRATION AND POSITION SENSE

128-Hz tuning fork.

HOW TO EXAMINE VIBRATION AND POSITION SENSE

Vibration Sense

1. Inform the patient that you will be using a vibrating ("buzzing") tuning fork to determine how well he or she feels this sensation.
2. It is helpful to start by making sure that the patient understands the definition of the sensation of the vibrating tuning fork as compared to the sensation of the nonvibrating tuning fork. To do this, have the patient keep his or her eyes open and strike the tuning fork (on your other hand) so that a moderate degree of vibration occurs. While holding the stem of the tuning fork between your thumb and index

finger, place the base of the tuning fork on an area where you would expect most patients to be able to feel it, such as on the wrist or forehead. Say to the patient, "This is vibration" (or "buzzing"), and, then, keeping the tuning fork on the patient, stop it from vibrating and say, "This is no vibration" (or "no buzzing"). Once you are convinced that the patient understands the ground rules of the test, proceed to testing vibratory sense.

3. Ask the patient to close his or her eyes.
4. Strike the tuning fork so that a slight degree of vibration occurs and, while holding the stem of the tuning fork between your thumb and index finger, place the base of the tuning fork on the distal phalanx of the patient's large toe and ask if he or she feels vibration (or "buzzing") or no vibration (or "no buzzing").
5. If the patient states that he or she can feel the slightly vibrating tuning fork, confirm that the patient actually felt the vibration by performing the same test but, this time, stop the tuning fork from vibrating before placing it on the patient's large toe. Again ask the patient if he or she feels vibration or no vibration. If the patient appropriately describes this as "no vibration," then the patient's (normal) ability to feel the slightly vibrating tuning fork in that extremity (step 4) has been confirmed, and there is no need to proceed with further testing in that extremity.
6. Perform the same test as step 4 on the large toe of the patient's other foot.
7. If the patient is not able to feel the slightly vibrating tuning fork distally, repeat the process with higher amplitude vibrations (by striking the tuning fork more strongly) and see how strong the vibration needs to be before the patient can feel the tuning fork distally. Each time you hold the tuning fork to the patient, ask if he or she feels vibration (or "buzzing") or no vibration (or "no buzzing"). In addition, you can assess for the severity of the proximal extent of the vibratory loss by striking the tuning fork to a moderate level of vibration, then placing it over more proximal bony prominences (the dorsum of the foot, the medial or lateral malleolus, the anterior shin, the knee, or even the iliac crest) until the patient states that he or she can feel the vibration.
8. The same procedure can be performed, if necessary, in the upper extremities, starting in the distal finger joints. Vibratory sensation testing in the upper extremities should be performed particularly when significant vibration sense loss is found in the lower extremities.

Position Sense (Proprioception)

1. Inform the patient that you will be moving his or her big toe up ("toward the ceiling") or down ("toward the ground") and that you will be asking him or her to tell you in which direction you have just moved it. If the patient is lying in bed, "up" and "down" might not be so obvious, so it is helpful to clarify that "toward your head is up" and "toward me is down" if you are standing at the foot of the bed.
2. Ask the patient to close his or her eyes.
3. Start your examination by testing the toes. Hold the distal phalanx of the patient's large toe on the sides, with your thumb on one side and your index finger on the other side. Don't hold one finger on the top and the other on the bottom, because your pressure would then give the patient a clue to the direction the toe is moving.
4. While moving the patient's toe slightly upward or downward, ask the patient, "Am I moving your toe up or down?"

5. Repeat the same process a few times with the same toe until you are convinced that the patient consistently gives the correct response or is making errors.
6. Perform the same test on the large toe of the patient's other foot.
7. If the patient's responses are incorrect distally, proprioception should be checked more and more proximally by checking the patient's ability to detect up and down movements of the proximal phalanx or the ankle or even the knee.
8. The same procedure can be performed, if necessary, in the upper extremities, starting in the distal finger joints. Position testing in the upper extremities should be performed particularly when significant position sense loss is found in the lower extremities.

NORMAL FINDINGS
Vibration Sense

Normally, patients should be able to feel the vibration from a slightly vibrating tuning fork in the distal toes and fingers. Use your perception of the vibrating tuning fork as you hold it on the patient to help guide what you think the neurologically healthy patient should be able to feel. The ability to detect vibration in the distal lower extremities does diminish with age, however, so neurologically healthy elderly patients may be expected to have at least a mild loss of vibration sensation in the toes, as compared to younger patients, even in the absence of sensory complaints or any clinically relevant nerve or spinal cord dysfunction.

Position Sense (Proprioception)

Normally, patients should be able to correctly detect the direction of small upward and downward movements in the toes and fingers. Proprioceptive sensation as tested clinically does not seem to significantly diminish with age.

ABNORMAL FINDINGS
Vibration Sense

• The inability to feel the vibration from a slightly vibrating tuning fork in the toes is abnormal in nonelderly patients, and the inability to feel a moderately vibrating tuning fork is abnormal in elderly patients. Report the patient's vibratory loss as mild, moderate, or severe. This can be described in several ways depending on the severity of the finding, such as "There is mild vibratory loss in the toes" or "There is severe vibratory loss up to the knees." Generally, the more severe the vibratory loss, the more likely the finding is to be clinically significant.
• Abnormal vibratory sensation in the lower extremities mainly suggests the presence of a peripheral neuropathy (sensory polyneuropathy), dysfunction of multiple lumbar nerve roots (lumbosacral polyradiculopathy), or a process within the spinal cord (myelopathy) at any level affecting the posterior columns. As with any examination finding, you would need to synthesize the findings from the history and the rest of the examination to try to distinguish between these possibilities.
• Vibratory loss in the upper extremities and the lower extremities suggests a severe polyneuropathy or a cervical myelopathy.

Position Sense

• The inability to correctly detect the direction of small upward or downward movements of the toes is abnormal and consistent with proprioceptive dysfunction; this is seen mainly in the clinical setting of a severe peripheral polyneuropathy or from spinal cord dysfunction (myelopathy) at any level affecting the posterior columns.

- Position sense loss in both the upper and the lower extremities suggests a severe sensory polyneuropathy or a cervical myelopathy.

ADDITIONAL POINTS

- The method of vibratory sense testing described here is different than the way many physicians perform the test. Many clinicians are taught to hold the vibrating tuning fork to the toe and ask the patient to let them know when the vibration has died down—this method takes too much time and runs the risk of the patient and physician becoming habituated to the sensory stimulus and bored.

- Assessing vibration sense routinely provides a better idea of the normal range of ability to detect vibration sense in the toes and the normal mild reduction in this ability with age. In addition, grading vibratory loss from mild to moderate to severe is subjective and is aided by testing lots of patients.

- Testing for position sense is not a substitute for testing vibration sense, because vibratory loss is a more sensitive and early symptom of sensory nerve or posterior column dysfunction than is position sense.

- Severe loss of vibration and position sense can also be seen as a result of dysfunction of the dorsal root ganglion cells (sensory neuronopathies); in these patients, loss of proprioception is often quite severe and can lead to the upper extremities assuming abnormal postures when the eyes are closed (called *pseudoathetosis*).

- Vibration and position sense can theoretically be affected by lesions above the cord, such as the thalamus or the parietal cortex. In practice, however, these tests are most helpful in diagnosing spinal cord or peripheral nerve dysfunction. When testing vibration and position sense, it's best to concentrate more on detecting the proximal-distal extent of loss than side-to-side differences.

- Asymmetric loss of posterior column sensation should be sought, however, when a hemi-spinal cord process is suspected (Brown-Séquard syndrome). In this syndrome, diminished posterior column sensation would be expected on the same side as weakness but contralateral to the side of pinprick sensation loss (see Chapter 51, Examination of the Patient with a Suspected Spinal Cord Problem).

Chapter 31

EXAMINATION OF CORTICAL SENSATION

PURPOSE

The purpose of the examination of cortical sensation is mainly to see if there is evidence for a lesion involving the nondominant (usually the right) parietal cortex.

WHEN TO EXAMINE CORTICAL SENSATION

Cortical sensation does not need to be assessed routinely. Examination of cortical sensation may be helpful, however, in situations in which there is a question of whether a patient's symptoms are due to a right hemisphere (cortical) process as opposed to a spinal cord or peripheral process. The finding of cortical sensory abnormalities in these situations, in the absence of significant gross loss to the primary sensory modalities, would be further evidence of a hemispheric (cortical) localization.

NEUROANATOMY OF CORTICAL SENSATION

Cortical sensation refers to sensation that requires some processing by the cortex to discriminate one stimulus from another. The cortical sensory modalities (described in sections below) include graphesthesia, stereognosis, and the ability to perceive the presence of bilateral simultaneous sensory stimuli. These cortical sensory functions are in contrast to the primary sensory modalities (such as pinprick and vibration) for which there are specific peripheral receptors and that don't require much further cortical integration.

EQUIPMENT NEEDED TO TEST CORTICAL SENSATION

- For graphesthesia: none
- For stereognosis: a few coins of different denominations
- For testing bilateral simultaneous stimulation: none

HOW TO EXAMINE CORTICAL SENSATION

Graphesthesia

1. Ask the patient to close his eyes and tell him you'll be writing a number on his hand and he should tell you what the number is.
2. Write any one-digit number on the palm of the patient's hand using your finger or a dull object like the cap of a pen and ask the patient what number it is. This may be repeated using a different number to confirm the accuracy of the patient's responses. It's helpful to "erase" the previous stimulus by rubbing the patient's palm with your hand between stimuli.
3. Repeat the same on the other hand.

Stereognosis

1. Ask the patient to close her eyes and tell her you'll be placing an object into her hand and she should try to tell you what it is.

2. Place a coin of any denomination in the patient's hand and ask her to identify it. Inform the patient that she can manipulate the object in her hand but should only use the one hand. If necessary, repeat this using a different (or even the same) coin to better assess the accuracy of the response.
3. Repeat the same on the other hand.

Bilateral Simultaneous Stimulation

Testing for extinction on double simultaneous stimulation can be performed with any sensory stimulus, as long as the same stimuli are used on both sides. The most common sensory modalities used to test for extinction are visual fields and gross touch.

To test bilateral simultaneous visual stimulation:

1. Begin as you would normally to check visual fields (see Chapter 13, Visual Field Examination): Stand directly across from the patient and ask the patient to look directly at your eyes.
2. Hold your left hand up so that you have one, two, or five fingers in the patient's right visual field and ask the patient to tell you how many fingers you're holding up (while he or she is still looking only at your eyes). Put your left hand down when you're done.
3. Then test the patient's left visual field alone by holding up your right hand with one, two, or five fingers. Put your right hand down when you're done.
4. Last, hold both hands up so that you're testing the patient's right and left visual fields at the same time (still with the patient looking only at your eyes). It's probably best to hold one finger up with one of your hands and two fingers up with your other hand. Ask the patient how many fingers you're holding up.

To test bilateral simultaneous touch:

1. Ask the patient to close his eyes and tell him you'll be touching him with your hands and that he should indicate which side you touch: left, right, or both.
2. Touch the patient's right arm with your left hand and listen for the patient's response.
3. Touch the patient's left arm with your right hand and listen for the response.
4. Finally, touch both of the patient's arms simultaneously with both of your hands and listen for the patient's response.

NORMAL FINDINGS

In the absence of significant cutaneous loss to the primary sensory modalities, patients should normally be able to identify a number drawn on each palm (graphesthesia), identify the denomination of individual coins in their hands (stereognosis), and recognize that the right and left extremities are being touched simultaneously. In the absence of a visual field deficit (hemianopsia), patients should normally be able to count fingers in both the right and the left visual fields simultaneously.

ABNORMAL FINDINGS

Graphesthesia

If there is normal cutaneous sensation to the primary sensory modalities, the inability to correctly identify a number drawn on the palm with the eyes closed is abnormal (agraphesthesia). An abnormality on this test is most likely to be of clinical significance when there is unilateral dysfunction, especially on the left hand; in this situation, the finding is suggestive of contralateral (i.e., right, nondominant) parietal cortical dysfunction.

Stereognosis

If there is normal cutaneous sensation to the primary sensory modalities, the inability to correctly identify the denomination of individual coins in the hand is abnormal (astereognosis). Similar to the test for graphesthesia, an abnormality on this test is most likely to be of significance when there is unilateral dysfunction on the left hand, suggestive of right parietal cortical dysfunction.

Bilateral Simultaneous Stimulation

In the absence of a hemianopsia, the inability to count fingers on one side when the examiner is holding fingers in both fields simultaneously is abnormal. In the absence of significant cutaneous loss to the primary sensory modalities, feeling that only one side of the body is being touched when in fact both sides are being touched is also abnormal. In either of these situations, the patient is said to have *extinction* of the stimulus on the side that he or she doesn't recognize. This would be reported as, "There was extinction on double simultaneous visual [or tactile] stimulation." Similar to the other cortical sensory tests, extinction is most commonly seen due to right (nondominant) parietal cortical dysfunction, in which the finding would be extinction of the left-sided stimulus.

ADDITIONAL POINTS

- There's no reason to test cortical sensation when the examination has already disclosed significant sensory dysfunction on one side, because any abnormal findings could be explained by the loss of primary sensation.
- When testing graphesthesia, even patients without cortical dysfunction sometimes have difficulty correctly identifying the number "4," probably because there are different ways to write it.

Chapter 32

ROMBERG TESTING

PURPOSE

The purpose of testing for the Romberg sign is to assess proprioceptive (position sense) function in the lower extremities.

WHEN TO PERFORM THE ROMBERG TEST

Romberg testing is quickly and easily performed, and it should be included during most neurologic examinations. It should be performed particularly on all patients who have a complaint of balance or gait dysfunction or falls, in patients with neuropathies, or in any other patient in whom proprioceptive dysfunction is suspected.

NEUROANATOMY (PATHOPHYSIOLOGY) OF ROMBERG TESTING

Assuming that there is enough strength to stand, the ability to maintain a stable upright stance depends on the intactness of two neurologic mechanisms:
- Balance (cerebellar and vestibular function)
- Sensation (vision or proprioception) to tell you where your feet and legs are in relationship to the ground

Both mechanisms (balance and sensation) are needed to be stable when upright. When your eyes are open, vision alone is enough to give you the sensory component of the equation. When your eyes are closed, the only way to tell where your feet and legs are in relation to the ground is through proprioceptive (joint position) sense.

EQUIPMENT NEEDED FOR ROMBERG TESTING

None.

HOW TO PERFORM THE ROMBERG TEST

1. Ask the patient to stand with his or her eyes open and observe that the patient can stand without falling. It's not imperative that the feet be touching, but it is best to have the feet as close together as possible as long as the patient can still maintain the upward stance with his or her eyes open.
2. Ask the patient to close his or her eyes.
3. Observe whether the patient can remain standing or will fall with his or her eyes closed. You don't need to observe for long, approximately 5 seconds at most.
4. If the patient would clearly fall without your assistance, help the patient avoid falling. If the patient sways but appears to be able to maintain balance, try to avoid assisting the patient unless it is clear that a fall is imminent. In other words, attempt to observe the patient's response; try not to be too quick to assume the patient will fall, but don't let the patient fall!

NORMAL FINDINGS

Normally, patients can stand with their eyes open and remain upright when their eyes are closed.

ABNORMAL FINDINGS

- The abnormal finding on the Romberg test is the Romberg sign itself. Patients with a Romberg sign are able to stand without falling with their eyes open but are unsteady and tend to fall soon after their eyes are closed.
- The finding of a Romberg sign suggests impairment of joint position (proprioceptive) sensation in the lower extremities. This is because patients with poor or absent proprioceptive sensation lose the entire sensory component of their ability to maintain the upright stance when their eyes are closed.
- The impairment of proprioceptive sensation suggested by a Romberg sign could be due to peripheral neuropathy or posterior column dysfunction within the spinal cord. When a Romberg sign is seen, it is likely that other signs of this dysfunction will also have been found, such as severe vibratory loss in the lower extremities and abnormal position sense testing in the toes or feet (see Chapter 30, Examination of Vibration and Position Sensation). If the proprioceptive dysfunction is severe enough, patients with a Romberg sign might even have the finding of a sensory ataxia on gait testing (see Chapter 39, Examination of Gait).
- Patients who sway and catch themselves, particularly at the hips, but regain balance and avoid falling while keeping their eyes closed, do not have a Romberg sign and, in fact, have shown you that they have excellent proprioception.

ADDITIONAL POINTS

- Although often reported as present (because of inaccurately interpreting the patient's swaying and catching him- or herself as a Romberg sign), the Romberg sign is actually an uncommon finding, because dysfunction of proprioceptive sensation severe enough to cause a Romberg sign is rare.
- Some patients give a history that implies the same information about proprioceptive dysfunction that a Romberg sign does. Patients who describe unsteadiness or falling in situations in which they stand with their eyes closed (such as when walking to the bathroom at night or when standing in the shower) are describing a self-tested Romberg sign, and they are likely to have proprioceptive dysfunction as the cause of their symptoms, regardless of whether they have a Romberg sign on examination.

Cerebellar Examination

Chapter 33

APPROACH TO THE CEREBELLAR EXAMINATION

PURPOSE

The purpose of testing cerebellar function is to look for evidence of a lesion involving the cerebellum or the cerebellar pathways.

WHEN TO PERFORM THE CEREBELLAR EXAMINATION

Cerebellar function should be examined in all patients as part of a standard neurologic examination. This should include the finger-to-nose maneuver (see Chapter 34, Testing of Upper Extremity Cerebellar Function) and observation of gait (see Chapter 39, Examination of Gait). Other tests of cerebellar function, such as rapid alternating movements or testing for rebound, should be performed when there is a clinical suspicion for a cerebellar abnormality and are discussed in Chapter 34, Testing of Upper Extremity Cerebellar Function, and Chapter 35, Testing of Lower Extremity Cerebellar Function.

NEUROANATOMY OF THE CEREBELLUM

The function of the cerebellum is to coordinate movements. The midline of the cerebellum (the vermis) is primarily involved in truncal balance and gait. The lateral parts of the cerebellum (the two cerebellar hemispheres) coordinate the movements of the ipsilateral extremities. In other words, the left cerebellar hemisphere coordinates the left arm and leg, and the right cerebellar hemisphere coordinates the right arm and leg.

There are also pathways to and from the cerebellum that travel through the cerebral hemispheres and the brainstem; these cerebellar pathways in the internal capsule and the base of the pons coordinate the contralateral extremities. In other words, the cerebellar-destined fibers located within the left internal capsule or left pons are involved in coordination of the right arm and right leg.

EQUIPMENT NEEDED TO EXAMINE CEREBELLAR FUNCTION

None.

HOW TO EXAMINE CEREBELLAR FUNCTION

Examination of upper extremity cerebellar function, including testing finger-to-nose, rapid alternating movements, and rebound, is described in Chapter

34, Testing of Upper Extremity Cerebellar Function. Examination of lower extremity cerebellar function, including heel-to-shin testing, is described in Chapter 35, Testing of Lower Extremity Cerebellar Function. The examination of gait and tandem gait is described in Chapter 39, Examination of Gait.

NORMAL FINDINGS

Patients whose motor and sensory functions are intact are able to smoothly and accurately perform the finger-to-nose and heel-to-shin maneuvers, are able to rapidly and accurately perform alternating movements in the hands, and have a stable and narrow-based gait.

ABNORMAL FINDINGS

Abnormal findings on cerebellar testing can be generally divided into the cerebellar abnormalities seen on examination of gait and the abnormalities seen on examination of the extremities.

Gait

- The abnormal finding on examination of gait due to cerebellar dysfunction is called *gait ataxia*, which is characterized by a wide-based, unsteady gait (sometimes with inability to walk at all because of the severe unsteadiness) and inability to perform tandem gait (see Chapter 39, Examination of Gait).
- Gait ataxia can be seen due to any lesion of the cerebellum in the midline (vermis) or in the hemispheres. Cerebellar vermis lesions tend to produce gait ataxia without significant extremity findings. Cerebellar hemisphere lesions, on the other hand, typically produce extremity findings (see Extremities) as well as gait ataxia. When patients with an ataxic gait tend to veer or fall consistently toward one side, the side that they veer toward is likely the side of the cerebellar hemisphere lesion.

Extremities

- The main type of abnormality seen on examination of the extremities due to cerebellar dysfunction is incoordination of the extremity.
- On the finger-to-nose or the heel-to-shin tests, findings of cerebellar dysfunction manifest as clumsiness in performance of the maneuver, usually with some side-to-side wavering of the extremity (including movements at the shoulder or hip) throughout its attempt to reach its target. This is cerebellar ataxia, which is probably better referred to as *appendicular ataxia* to distinguish it from the finding of gait ataxia described in Gait.
- There are many other names for the clumsiness seen in the extremities due to cerebellar disease, including *dysmetria*. Although dysmetria probably more accurately refers to the overshoot or undershoot of the target seen in cerebellar disease, in practice the term *dysmetria* is used as a generic term synonymous with appendicular ataxia to describe any cerebellar-type clumsiness during the finger-to-nose or the heel-to-shin tests. In fact, *dysmetria* seems to be the preferred term by most clinicians to describe any clumsiness seen during the finger-to-nose or the heel-to-shin tests attributed to cerebellar dysfunction.
- Asymmetric or unilateral dysmetria (i.e., appendicular ataxia) in the arm or leg, or both, in the absence of any weakness suggests a cerebellar hemisphere lesion ipsilateral to the side of the clumsiest extremities.

TABLE 33-1 Summary of the Lesions within the Cerebellum or Its Pathways That May Cause Incoordination on Examination

Location of Lesion	Area of Body Where Coordination Is Affected
Vermis (midline)	Trunk (gait)
Left cerebellar hemisphere	Left extremities
Right cerebellar hemisphere	Right extremities
Left posterior limb of internal capsule or the left base of pons	Right extremities; also with mild right-sided weakness (*ataxic-hemiparesis*)
Right posterior limb of internal capsule or the right base of pons	Left extremities; also with mild left-sided weakness (*ataxic-hemiparesis*)

- Other abnormal findings in the extremities that may be seen on cerebellar testing include difficulty performing rapid, alternating movements (*dysdiadochokinesia*) and *rebound* in the arms. These findings, which also occur ipsilateral to the cerebellar hemispheric lesion, are described in further detail in Chapter 34, Testing of Upper Extremity Cerebellar Function.
- Weakness does not occur due to dysfunction of the cerebellum, whether in the cerebellar hemispheres or the vermis. Sometimes, however, patients with mild weakness in an extremity also have what appears to be cerebellar dysmetria in the same extremity (i.e., the mild weakness doesn't seem to be severe enough to explain the dysmetria). In such cases (called *ataxic-hemiparesis*), the lesion may be in the contralateral posterior limb of the internal capsule or the pons.
- Table 33–1 summarizes the effect of lesions within the cerebellum or its pathways that may cause incoordination on cerebellar testing.
- Cerebellar disease may also cause tremor. The term *intention tremor*, however, is sometimes used to describe cerebellar dysmetria, which is not really a tremor at all, but rather, as described previously, is clumsiness and wavering in an attempt to reach a target. True tremors due to cerebellar pathway disease are, however, usually worse with action and may be coarse. A rhythmic tremor of the head or trunk, or both, can also occur due to cerebellar disease and is known as *titubation*.

ADDITIONAL POINTS

Much of the terminology used to describe cerebellar findings on examination is vague and ambiguous. Try to avoid the term *intention tremor* to describe clumsiness during the finger-to-nose and heel-to-shin maneuvers, as this term can be confused with other true tremors of cerebellar or noncerebellar (see Chapter 46, Examination of the Patient with a Movement Disorder) etiologies. Sticking to the terminology recommended here (e.g., dysmetria, appendicular ataxia) is less confusing.

Chapter 34

TESTING OF UPPER EXTREMITY CEREBELLAR FUNCTION

PURPOSE

The purpose of testing upper extremity cerebellar function is to look for evidence of a lesion involving the cerebellar hemispheres or the cerebellar pathways.

WHEN TO TEST UPPER EXTREMITY CEREBELLAR FUNCTION

The finger-to-nose maneuver, a simple screening test of upper extremity cerebellar function, should be performed on all patients as part of a standard neurologic examination. Other tests of upper extremity cerebellar function, such as rapid alternating movements or testing for rebound, don't need to be performed routinely. These additional tests of cerebellar function should be performed when the possibility of cerebellar dysfunction is suggested by the history or you need to look for additional confirmation of cerebellar dysfunction when an abnormality is suggested on the finger-to-nose test.

NEUROANATOMY OF UPPER EXTREMITY CEREBELLAR FUNCTION

The basic relevant neuroanatomy of the cerebellum and its pathways is discussed in Chapter 33, Approach to the Cerebellar Examination. The left cerebellar hemisphere coordinates the left arm (and leg), and the right cerebellar hemisphere coordinates the right arm (and leg). Table 33–1 summarizes the lesions within the cerebellum or its pathways that may cause incoordination on examination.

EQUIPMENT NEEDED TO TEST UPPER EXTREMITY CEREBELLAR FUNCTION

None.

HOW TO EXAMINE UPPER EXTREMITY CEREBELLAR FUNCTION

Finger-to-Nose Examination

1. Ask the patient to "make a pointer" with his or her index finger.
2. Ask the patient to touch his or her nose with that index finger.
3. Hold your index finger directly in front of the patient, at nearly an arm's length away from him or her, and ask the patient to touch your index finger.
4. Ask the patient to repeat the process back and forth a few times, moving his or her index finger between the tip of the patient's nose and your index finger, as smoothly as possible.
5. Repeat the same process with the patient's other arm.

Rapid Alternating Movements (Diadochokinesia)

1. Show the patient what you will be asking him or her to do by holding one of your hands stationary with its palm up, then rapidly clap your other

hand on the stationary hand, alternately turning the moving hand palm side up or palm side down (i.e., alternating pronation and supination), alternating between each clap.

2. Ask the patient to perform this maneuver on one side while you watch for a few seconds. If you suspect that the patient might be ataxic on a particular side, it is probably best to have the patient begin the test by moving the good side and holding the other (potentially ataxic) arm stationary.

3. Then ask the patient to perform the same maneuver with the opposite hands (i.e., keeping the other hand stationary) while you observe for a few seconds.

Rebound

1. Ask the patient to hold both arms directly in front of him or her, palm side down.

2. Tell the patient to try to keep the arms in the same position without moving and specifically to resist your attempt to push the arms down.

3. Using both of your hands, press down on the dorsum of both of your patient's hands while the patient resists that force, and then let go.

4. Observe the response of the patient's arms after you let go of them.

NORMAL FINDINGS

Finger-to-Nose Examination

Normally, the patient should be able to perform the finger-to-nose maneuver smoothly and accurately with each arm, and there should be no significant asymmetry between the two arms.

Rapid Alternating Movements (Diadochokinesia)

Patients should normally be able to rapidly clap one hand on the other, alternating supination and pronation of the moving hand, fairly smoothly and accurately on each side. Some neurologically normal patients, however, perform this maneuver slightly less smoothly when the nondominant hand is the moving hand.

Test for Rebound

Normally, the patient's arms should rebound slightly upward when you release your downward pressure on them. This slight rebound should be symmetric, however, and the patient's arms should rapidly return to their straight, forward position.

ABNORMAL FINDINGS

Finger-to-Nose Examination

- Clumsiness of an arm during the finger-to-nose maneuver is abnormal. Clumsiness due to cerebellar dysfunction usually manifests as side-to-side wavering of the arm (including movements at the shoulder) throughout its attempt to reach its target; this is referred to as *dysmetria* or *appendicular ataxia* (or simply *ataxia*). See Chapter 33, Approach to the Cerebellar Examination, for a discussion of the terminology describing cerebellar dysfunction.

- Assuming the patient's arm is strong (cerebellar hemisphere lesions do not cause weakness), clumsiness during the finger-to-nose maneuver on one side suggests cerebellar hemisphere dysfunction ipsilateral to the side of the clumsy extremity.

- When patients with mild weakness in an extremity also have what appears to be significant cerebellar dysmetria in the same extremity (and the subtle weakness doesn't seem to be severe enough to explain the dysmetria), the lesion may be in the contralateral posterior limb of the internal capsule or the pons. This is called an *ataxic-hemiparesis* (see Table 33–1).

Rapid Alternating Movements (Diadochokinesia)

- Inability to rapidly, smoothly, and accurately perform rapid alternating movements in the upper extremities is abnormal and is called *dysdiadochokinesia*. As noted in the section Normal Finding, however, a mild asymmetry in ability to perform this test (worse in the nondominant hand) may not be abnormal.
- In the absence of any weakness, a significant problem performing rapid alternating movements on one side (dysdiadochokinesia) is suggestive of cerebellar hemisphere dysfunction ipsilateral to the side of the clumsy extremity.
- This test can be particularly affected by weakness, so in the presence of any weakness in an extremity, difficulty with rapid alternating movements can be a nonspecific finding.

Test for Rebound

Rebound, manifested by a loss of the normal check mechanism when you release your downward pressure on the patient's arm, is abnormal. The abnormal side rebounds significantly upward and then bounces down and up several times, as if it is held by a loose spring, before finally settling back to the straight, forward position. The finding of rebound, like the finding of dysmetria or dysdiadochokinesia, is ipsilateral to the abnormal cerebellar hemisphere.

ADDITIONAL POINTS

- The patient's eyes should be open throughout the cerebellar examination, including during the finger-to-nose maneuver. No additional information regarding cerebellar function is learned by having the patient's eyes closed.
- During the finger-to-nose maneuver, it is usually not necessary to give the patient a variable target by moving your finger to different positions, but occasionally this is helpful to bring out dysmetria that was not otherwise evident (or to further prove that the patient's coordination is good). To do this, move your finger to a different position—always at approximately the same distance from the patient (i.e., slightly less than an arm's length away)—when the patient brings his or her finger to his or her nose, and then keep your finger stationary in the new position until the patient brings his or her finger to yours.
- The bounciness of an arm on the side of cerebellar dysfunction, as seen on the test for rebound, may occasionally be suggested earlier in the examination when the patient brings the arms into position when testing drift.

Chapter 35

TESTING OF LOWER EXTREMITY CEREBELLAR FUNCTION

PURPOSE

The purpose of testing lower extremity cerebellar function is to look for evidence of a lesion involving the cerebellar hemispheres or the cerebellar pathways.

WHEN TO TEST LOWER EXTREMITY CEREBELLAR FUNCTION

The heel-to-shin maneuver, a simple screening test of lower extremity cerebellar function, should be performed on most patients as part of a standard neurologic examination. When cerebellar dysfunction is not suggested by the history or the preceding parts of the examination, however, it's reasonable to stop the examination of cerebellar function after the (normal) finger-to-nose maneuver is completed. When there is a clinical suspicion for cerebellar dysfunction or to look for additional confirmation of cerebellar dysfunction when an abnormality is suggested on the upper extremity cerebellar examination (see Chapter 34, Testing of Upper Extremity Cerebellar Function), lower extremity cerebellar function should be tested.

Examination of gait, which should be a routine part of the neurologic examination, is discussed in Chapter 39, Examination of Gait.

NEUROANATOMY OF LOWER EXTREMITY CEREBELLAR FUNCTION

The basic relevant neuroanatomy of the cerebellum and its pathways is discussed in Chapter 33, Approach to the Cerebellar Examination. The left cerebellar hemisphere coordinates the left leg (and arm), and the right cerebellar hemisphere coordinates the right leg (and arm). Table 33–1 summarizes the lesions within the cerebellum or its pathways that may cause incoordination on cerebellar testing.

EQUIPMENT NEEDED TO TEST LOWER EXTREMITY CEREBELLAR FUNCTION

None.

HOW TO EXAMINE LOWER EXTREMITY CEREBELLAR FUNCTION

The main test of cerebellar function performed in the lower extremities is the *heel-to-shin examination:*

1. With the patient sitting in a chair or lying in bed, ask the patient to place one of his or her heels up on the knee of the opposite leg. The heel-to-shin maneuver needs to be performed without the patient using his or her arms for assistance.

2. Then ask the patient to smoothly move the heel all the way (straight) down the other leg to the ankle, keeping his or her heel on the anterior shin bone of the other leg throughout the maneuver.

3. Once the patient's heel has gone down to the ankle, ask the patient to move his or her heel back up the leg to the knee, again keeping the heel on the shin of the other leg.
4. Repeat the same maneuver with the other leg.

NORMAL FINDINGS

Normally, the patient should be able to perform the heel-to-shin maneuver smoothly and accurately with each leg, and there should be no significant asymmetry between the two sides.

ABNORMAL FINDINGS

- Clumsiness of a leg during the heel-to-shin test is abnormal. Clumsiness due to cerebellar dysfunction usually manifests as side-to-side wavering of the leg (including movements at the hip) throughout its attempt to reach its target; this is referred to as *dysmetria* or *appendicular ataxia* (or simply *ataxia*) (see Chapter 33, Approach to the Cerebellar Examination).
- Assuming the patient's leg is strong (cerebellar hemisphere lesions do not cause weakness), clumsiness during the heel-to-shin maneuver on one side suggests cerebellar hemisphere dysfunction ipsilateral to the side of the clumsy leg.
- As in the upper extremities, when patients with mild weakness in the leg also have what appears to be cerebellar dysmetria in the same leg (and the subtle weakness doesn't seem to be severe enough to explain the dysmetria), the lesion may be in the contralateral posterior limb of the internal capsule or the pons. This is called an *ataxic-hemiparesis* (see Table 33–1).

ADDITIONAL POINTS

Because of the mechanics of the test, the ability to perform the heel-to-shin maneuver (even in the absence of cerebellar dysfunction) is particularly affected by weakness (especially hip flexion), body habitus, and hip problems, so keep this in mind when performing and interpreting this examination element.

Chapter 36

APPROACH TO REFLEX TESTING

PURPOSE

The purpose of testing reflexes is to localize neurologic pathology to the central or the peripheral nervous system by looking for evidence of upper motor neuron or lower motor neuron (or peripheral sensory nerve) dysfunction.

WHEN TO TEST REFLEXES

Testing of muscle stretch reflexes and testing for the Babinski sign should be performed on all patients as part of a standard neurologic examination.

NEUROANATOMY OF REFLEXES

The muscle stretch reflexes and the Babinski sign are spinal reflexes. In both of these reflexes, the stimulus sends an afferent (sensory) impulse up a sensory nerve into the dorsal root of the spinal cord, which completes the reflex arc by ultimately synapsing on motor neurons within the spinal cord, causing an efferent (motor) response. The corticospinal tract (the upper motor neuron) has an inhibitory influence on the muscle stretch reflexes and the Babinski sign.

EQUIPMENT NEEDED TO TEST REFLEXES

- A reflex hammer to test muscle stretch reflexes (see Chapter 37, Examination of the Muscle Stretch Reflexes)
- A blunt object to test for the Babinski sign (see Chapter 38, Testing for the Babinski Response)

HOW TO TEST REFLEXES

See Chapter 37, Examination of the Muscle Stretch Reflexes, and Chapter 38, Testing for the Babinski Response, for testing discussion.

NORMAL FINDINGS

Normally, patients should have intact but not severely hyperactive muscle stretch reflexes. There should also be no Babinski sign in either foot.

ABNORMAL FINDINGS

There are two main kinds of abnormal findings that can be seen on reflex testing: findings due to the loss of the normal inhibitory influence of the upper motor neuron on the reflexes and findings due to lesions of the lower motor neuron or sensory nerve affecting the reflex arc itself.

TABLE 36-1 Interpretation of Abnormal Reflexes

Reflex Finding	Localization of Dysfunction Primarily Suggested
Hyperactive muscle stretch reflexes	
Diffuse hyperreflexic muscle stretch reflexes	Bilateral hemisphere or brainstem
	Bilateral upper cervical spinal cord
Unilateral hyperreflexic muscle stretch reflexes	Unilateral (contralateral) hemisphere or brainstem
	Unilateral (ipsilateral) spinal cord
Hyperreflexic muscle stretch reflexes only in the legs	Thoracic spinal cord (cervical cord still possible)
Hypoactive muscle stretch reflexes	
Diffuse areflexic (or severely hyporeflexic) muscle stretch reflexes	Polyneuropathy or polyradiculopathy
Distal absence of muscle stretch reflexes (e.g., absent ankle jerks)	Polyneuropathy
Single absent muscle stretch reflex	Radiculopathy
Babinski sign	
Bilateral Babinski signs	Bilateral hemisphere, brainstem, or spinal cord
Unilateral Babinski sign	Unilateral (contralateral) hemisphere or brainstem
	Unilateral (ipsilateral) spinal cord

Abnormalities due to Upper Motor Neuron (Corticospinal Tract) Dysfunction: Hyperreflexia and the Babinski Sign

- The corticospinal tracts are the upper motor neurons. Abnormalities on reflex testing that occur as a result of corticospinal tract dysfunction are called *upper motor neuron signs*, and they can occur due to any cause of corticospinal tract dysfunction anywhere along their course, from their origin as neurons in the motor cortex to their descent in the spinal cord. These upper motor neuron signs occur due to the loss of the normal inhibitory influence that the corticospinal tract has on the muscle stretch reflexes, which therefore become hyperactive (*hyperreflexic*), and the loss of the normal inhibitory influence that the corticospinal tract has on the Babinski sign, which results.
- In addition to muscle stretch reflex hyperreflexia and the Babinski sign, other upper motor neuron findings can include *clonus* (a severe form of muscle stretch reflex hyperreflexia) and increased tone (stiffness) due to spasticity in the involved limbs (see Chapter 27, Examination of Tone). Upper motor neuron signs are usually, but not invariably, also accompanied by weakness in the involved extremities.

Abnormalities due to Dysfunction of the Reflex Arc Itself: Hyporeflexia

- Dysfunction of either the lower motor neuron (efferent) or sensory (afferent) components of the reflex arc may cause diminished (hyporeflexic) or absent (areflexic) muscle stretch reflexes in the involved extremities. Depending on the cause and severity of the process, the diminished reflexes may be accompanied by weakness (due to lower motor neuron dysfunction), sensory loss, or even hypotonia in the involved extremity.

- Table 36–1 summarizes the potential localizations suggested by the distribution of abnormal reflexes. More information regarding the interpretation of these abnormal reflexes can be found in Chapter 37, Examination of the Muscle Stretch Reflexes, and Chapter 38, Testing for the Babinski Response.

EXAMINATION OF THE MUSCLE STRETCH REFLEXES

PURPOSE

The purpose of testing muscle stretch reflexes is to localize neurologic pathology to the central or the peripheral nervous system by looking for evidence of upper motor neuron or lower motor neuron (or peripheral sensory nerve) dysfunction.

WHEN TO TEST THE MUSCLE STRETCH REFLEXES

Muscle stretch reflexes in the biceps, triceps, knees, and ankles should be examined in all patients as part of a routine neurologic examination. Testing for clonus in the ankles should be performed when hyperreflexia is seen in the lower extremities.

NEUROANATOMY OF THE MUSCLE STRETCH REFLEXES

The muscle spindles are sensory organs located within the muscles that sense muscle stretch (lengthening). Tapping a tendon with a reflex hammer causes a sudden muscle stretch that activates the muscle spindles. The muscle spindles send a sensory impulse to the spinal cord, which then synapses with motor neurons at that level of the spinal cord to initiate reflex contraction of the same muscle that was stretched. For example, tapping the left quadriceps tendon at the knee stretches the left quadriceps muscle (and its muscle spindles), initiating reflex contraction of the left quadriceps muscle, which is observed clinically as extension of the knee. The corticospinal tract—the upper motor neuron—has an inhibitory influence on the muscle stretch reflexes in the spinal cord.

EQUIPMENT NEEDED TO TEST THE MUSCLE STRETCH REFLEXES

- A reflex hammer.
- Any kind of reflex hammer will do, but reflexes are easier to obtain with a heavier hammer than the typical lightweight, tomahawk-style reflex hammer. Many neurologists prefer the Queen Square type of hammer, which consists of a rubber-rimmed disc on the end of a stick. Others, including the author, prefer a Tromner-style hammer, which is more "hammer-like" than the Queen Square hammer or the tomahawk. All reflex hammers are fairly inexpensive; go to a medical bookstore and pick out a hammer that you'll actually carry around and that works well for you.

HOW TO EXAMINE THE MUSCLE STRETCH REFLEXES

Routine Testing of Muscle Stretch Reflexes

1. It is easiest to test the reflexes with the patient sitting on the side of a bed or an examining table; however, the muscle stretch reflexes can also be tested with the patient lying in bed.

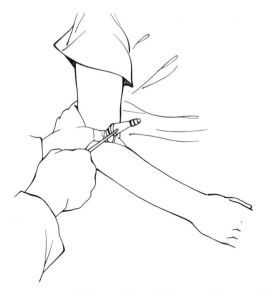

Figure 37–1 Testing the biceps reflex. Hold the patient's arm so that it is passively flexed and that your thumb is resting on the biceps tendon. Tap on your thumb with the reflex hammer.

2. Test the upper extremity reflexes before testing the lower extremity reflexes. It's also best to check the same reflex on each side before proceeding to the next muscle. In other words, start by testing the right biceps jerk, then test the left biceps jerk, then test the right triceps jerk, the left triceps jerk, and so forth.

3. Figures 37–1 through 37–4 illustrate and describe how to examine the major muscle stretch reflexes in the upper and lower extremities. Hold each limb in the optimal position for reflex testing for that muscle, as indicated in the figures. It's important to have the patient's limb as relaxed as possible (simply asking the patient to relax the muscle often helps).

4. Grade the reflex on a scale of 0 to 4, with 0 meaning the reflex is unobtainable and 4 meaning it is severely hyperreflexic. Table 37–1 summarizes the definition of the grading scale used for muscle stretch reflex testing. It is standard to report the grade as the number with a plus sign after it. The plus has no real meaning, but it is standard to write it that way. If you want, you can write the number without the plus, because there is no distinction between a 2, for example, and a 2+. Unlike muscle strength grading, a minus signs tends not to be used, so think of the reflex choices as only five grades (from 0 to 4), and choose the one grade that seems to fit best. Some clinicians prefer one more choice, however, between 0 and 1, called *trace*, meaning that there may be a suggestion of a slight reflex present, enough not to call it areflexic.

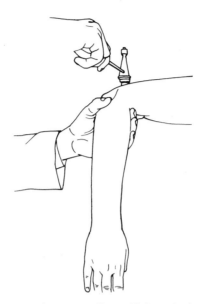

Figure 37–2 Testing the triceps reflex. Hold the patient's arm so that the upper arm is abducted at the shoulder and the arm is passively dangling at the elbow. Tap on the triceps tendon with the reflex hammer.

Testing Reflexes with Reinforcement

When a reflex seems unobtainable or is much diminished, it may be because the patient's muscle was not relaxed and the patient is inadvertently suppressing the reflex. In this situation, it is useful to try to distract the patient from the reflex task; this may bring out the reflex if it is really intact and is called *reinforcement of the reflex*. Several maneuvers are helpful to do this: One method of distraction is simply to ask the patient to "bite down" at the time you test the reflex; another maneuver is to ask the patient to make a tight fist with the opposite hand while you test the upper extremity reflex on the other side.

The following common maneuver is particularly helpful when testing lower extremity reflexes:

1. Instruct the patient to curl the fingers of each hand and lock the fingers together in front of him or her.
2. Ask the patient to pull the arms tight (still locked at the fingers) at the count of three.
3. Say "1, 2, 3, pull!" and tap on the lower extremity reflex with the hammer while the patient pulls the arms tight.

When a reflex is only readily obtained using one of these maneuvers but is difficult to obtain without the maneuver, it should be graded according to the grade with the maneuver, because the true reflex was brought out by the distraction. This can be reported, for example, as, "The biceps jerk was 2+ with reinforcement."

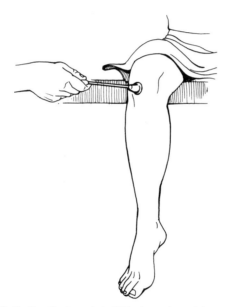

Figure 37–3 Testing the knee jerk. With the patient sitting and the legs dangling, tap on the quadriceps tendon (if the patient is lying in bed, lift the patient's thigh up slightly with your hand under the posterior thigh so that the leg is slightly passively flexed at the knee and relaxed, then tap on the patellar tendon).

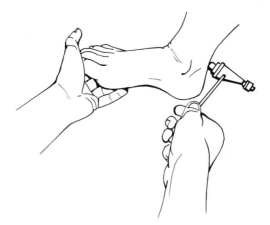

Figure 37–4 Testing the ankle jerk. Push the patient's foot slightly upward so that it is passively slightly dorsiflexed at the ankle, and then tap on the Achilles tendon.

TABLE 37-1 Grading of the Muscle Stretch Reflexes[a]

Grade	Definition	Comments
0	Absent reflex	No reflex, even with distracting maneuvers.
1+	Slight reflex	Reflex is definitely present, but diminished; possibly pathologic, depending on the clinical situation.
2+	Typical reflex	This is the average normal reflex, but 1+ and 3+ reflexes can also potentially be normal, depending on the clinical situation.
3+	Brisk reflex	Very brisk reflex; possibly pathologic, depending on the clinical situation.
4+	Very hyperactive reflex	Clearly pathologically hyperactive; 4+ in ankles implies that clonus is also present.

[a]See text for details of interpretation of possible reflex abnormalities.

Testing for Ankle Clonus

1. Hold the patient's posterior calf with one hand while you hold your other hand on the sole of the patient's foot.
2. Keeping the patient's leg stationary, abruptly (but not painfully) push the sole of the patient's foot upward.
3. Maintain upward pressure on the patient's foot, so that it stays forcefully (again, not painfully) dorsiflexed for a few seconds and observe the response.

NORMAL FINDINGS

Normally, muscle stretch reflexes should be present in the biceps, triceps, quadriceps (the patellar reflex or knee jerk), and the Achilles reflex (ankle jerk). These reflexes should be 1+, 2+, or 3+ and be reasonably symmetric on both sides. If ankle clonus is tested, there should be no more than a couple of beats of clonus seen.

There are some normal variations to be aware of, however. It is normal for some elderly patients to have diminished ankle jerks, even in the absence of symptoms of a polyneuropathy. Although variable, younger patients tend to have brisker reflexes than older patients, and reflexes are often brisker with anxiety. Last, triceps reflexes are sometimes harder to obtain than the other reflexes described.

ABNORMAL FINDINGS

Hyperreflexia

- Hyperreflexia of the muscle stretch reflexes is potentially abnormal. Because the corticospinal tract (the upper motor neuron) normally has an inhibitory influence on the reflexes, hyperreflexia—especially extreme hyperreflexia—of the muscle stretch reflexes suggests dysfunction of the corticospinal tract (in the brain, brainstem, or spinal cord) anywhere above the segment of the spinal cord that serves that reflex. Table 36-1 summarizes the lesion localizations suggested by different patterns of hyperreflexia.
- Although very hyperactive reflexes, such as sustained clonus (see following section, Clonus), are usually clearly pathologic, the normal patient-to-patient variation in reflexes makes it important to interpret reflexes only

TABLE 37–2 Spinal Root Levels Tested by the Muscle Stretch Reflexes

Reflex	Levels Involved
Biceps	C5, C6
Triceps	C7, C8
Quadriceps	L2, L3, L4
Achilles	S1

within the context of the clinical situation and not to overinterpret isolated reflex findings. The likelihood of significance of a reflex finding is greater when it was anticipated by the clinical history and the rest of the examination. For example, in the clinical setting of bilateral upper and lower extremity weakness and numbness due to a probable cervical spinal cord process (myelopathy), the finding of 3+ hyperreflexia would support that clinical localization. On the other hand, in a patient without motor or sensory symptoms, the finding of the same diffusely brisk reflexes would likely be a clinically nonsignificant finding and normal for that patient.

Clonus

Sustained ankle clonus is abnormal and is manifested by continuous rhythmic plantar flexion of the foot while the examiner holds the foot in a position to force dorsiflexion. Sustained clonus is simply extreme hyperreflexia, with the same implications as the finding of hyperreflexia described previously (see Hyperreflexia). Clonus can occur elsewhere, but it most commonly occurs at the ankle; it rarely can be seen when the patellar reflex is tested in patients who are markedly hyperreflexic at the knee.

Hyporeflexia

- Hyporeflexia of the muscle stretch reflexes is potentially abnormal, and absence of a muscle stretch reflex (areflexia) is usually abnormal. Decreased or absent muscle stretch reflexes suggest lower motor neuron or sensory nerve dysfunction at the level of the reflex tested, affecting the reflex arc. Table 36–1 summarizes the localizations suggested by different patterns of hyporeflexia. In general, diffuse or distal hyporeflexia or areflexia is most suggestive of a polyneuropathy, and solitary hyporeflexia or areflexia is most commonly seen due to individual nerve root dysfunction (radiculopathy).

- In the clinical setting of a suspected cervical or lumbar radiculopathy (see Chapter 47, Examination of the Patient with a Radiculopathy), the finding of a diminished or absent muscle stretch reflex is a particularly helpful sign in localization of the nerve root dysfunction. Table 37–2 summarizes the spinal root levels involved in producing the reflex arc for the four major muscle stretch reflexes. Hyporeflexia or areflexia of one of these reflexes in the clinical context of a probable radiculopathy in that extremity would suggest dysfunction of the nerve root involved in that reflex. For example, a patient with pain radiating down the posterior left leg who has an absent left ankle jerk (but all other reflexes are present) most likely has a left S1 radiculopathy.

ADDITIONAL POINTS

- A useful mnemonic to remember the root levels involved in the muscle stretch reflexes is *1,2,3,4,5,6,7,8* from bottom to top: the ankle jerk tests the S1 level; the knee jerk tests L2, L3, and L4; the biceps jerk tests C5 and C6; and the triceps jerk tests C7 and C8.

- Testing reflexes in all your patients undergoing a neurologic examination will give you the best feel of the normal variation of reflexes and help you decide what "normal," "hypoactive," or "hyperactive" is—although the clinical situation is always most important in deciding whether a reflex is pathologically brisk or diminished.

- The brachioradialis reflex is another C5, C6 reflex (similar to the biceps reflex). This can be tested by tapping on the insertion of the brachioradialis tendon on the dorsal lateral radius a couple of centimeters proximal to the wrist. Although usually obtainable, this reflex isn't as readily elicited as the other upper extremity reflexes, and for most clinical situations, it rarely adds much to the examination that wasn't already discovered by the biceps reflex.

- The muscle stretch reflexes are also commonly referred to as *deep tendon reflexes*. This terminology is not neuroanatomically accurate because the reflex tested is initiated by muscle stretch and not from the Golgi tendon organs; however, many clinical neurologists, including, admittedly, this author, still use the term. Use whatever terminology you like.

Chapter 38

TESTING FOR THE BABINSKI RESPONSE

PURPOSE

The purpose of testing for the Babinski response is to look for evidence of a lesion involving the corticospinal tract.

WHEN TO TEST FOR THE BABINSKI RESPONSE

Testing for the Babinski response should be performed on all patients as part of a standard neurologic examination.

NEUROANATOMY OF THE BABINSKI RESPONSE

The corticospinal tracts originate in the motor neurons of the cerebral cortex (the upper motor neurons) and descend into the opposite side of the spinal cord (see Chapter 24, Approach to the Motor Examination). The corticospinal tracts have an inhibitory influence on the Babinski sign; the inhibitory influence of an intact corticospinal tract suppresses the Babinski sign entirely.

EQUIPMENT NEEDED TO TEST THE BABINSKI RESPONSE

A blunt (preferably disposable) object, such as the bottom of a closed safety pin, a wooden stick, or a split tongue depressor.

HOW TO EXAMINE THE BABINSKI RESPONSE

1. Testing for the Babinski response can be performed with the patient sitting or lying down. The patient's foot should be relaxed.
2. With a blunt object, stroke the sole of one foot, starting near the heel and proceeding forward along the lateral sole. The maneuver should be performed in one smooth motion over 1 or 2 seconds. Observe the response (particularly the response of the big toe).
3. Perform the same test on the other foot.

NORMAL FINDINGS

Normally, stroking the bottom of the foot with a blunt object results in flexion of the toes. This normal finding can be reported as "no Babinski sign is present," "plantar responses are flexor bilaterally," or "the toes are downgoing bilaterally." Most neurologists seem to prefer the "downgoing toes" terminology for the normal response.

ABNORMAL FINDINGS

- The abnormal finding on Babinski testing is the Babinski sign itself. The Babinski sign consists of extension of the big toe after the sole of the foot is stroked; this can occur with or without fanning of the other toes (Fig. 38–1).
- The Babinski sign is an upper motor neuron sign; it can occur due to any cause of corticospinal tract dysfunction anywhere along its course, from its origin in the motor cortex to its descent in the spinal cord. The Babin-

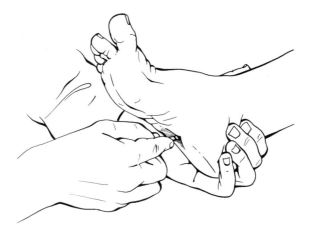

Figure 38–1 The Babinski sign: extension of the big toe after the sole of the foot is stroked.

ski sign occurs as a result of the loss of the normal inhibitory influence of the corticospinal tract. Localizations suggested by the presence of unilateral or bilateral Babinski signs are summarized in Table 36–1.

- The presence of a Babinski sign can be reported in several ways. It can be reported as a "Babinski sign," an "extensor plantar response," or an "upgoing toe." Most neurologists seem to prefer the "upgoing toe" terminology.
- The presence of a Babinski sign is always abnormal; however, the decision as to whether the response seen is truly a Babinski sign is not always so easy. It's not uncommon for patients to exhibit withdrawal to the plantar stimulus, consisting of dorsiflexion of the foot and toes, which can look like a Babinski sign. Babinski signs often consist of more subtle large toe dorsiflexion than the marked foot and toe dorsiflexion commonly seen due to withdrawal. Because the withdrawal reaction represents a ticklish response, repeating the stimulus after reassuring the patient and asking the patient to relax may help limit this reaction.

ADDITIONAL POINTS

- The Babinski sign is one of the most important signs in neurology. Its presence, even without other signs of upper motor neuron dysfunction, is an important clue to a corticospinal tract lesion; however, the Babinski sign, like any other finding, needs to be interpreted in the context of the patient's whole clinical picture.
- Many patients with Babinski signs have only large toe dorsiflexion as their abnormal response. You don't need to see fanning of the toes for the patient to have a Babinski sign.
- If the patient has difficulty relaxing the foot while you are performing the test, it's helpful to take the patient's mind off the task by asking a historical question or simply talking with the patient.

Gait Examination

EXAMINATION OF GAIT

PURPOSE

The main purpose of the examination of gait is to localize neurologic dysfunction by looking for characteristic patterns of gait abnormalities.

WHEN TO PERFORM THE GAIT EXAMINATION

Gait should be assessed in all patients in whom ambulation can be attempted as part of a standard neurologic examination. In patients who can attempt it safely, tandem gait should also be examined in most patients as part of a standard neurologic examination. Testing the patient's ability to walk on the heels or the toes needs only to be performed when weakness of foot dorsiflexion or plantar flexion is suspected.

NEUROANATOMY OF GAIT

Walking requires the coordinated effort of several neurologic structures and functions:

- The frontal lobes to generate the motor pathways to initiate gait
- Cerebellar (and vestibular) function for coordination and balance
- The basal ganglia for appropriate speed of movement
- Muscle strength to move the legs and to overcome gravity to remain upright
- Sensation, particularly proprioception, to know where the feet and legs are in space

EQUIPMENT NEEDED TO EXAMINE GAIT

None.

HOW TO EXAMINE GAIT

Gait

1. The gait can be tested with the patient's shoes on or off. If gait is tested outside the patient's room, it is best to have the patient wear shoes. In a patient without a suspicion for a significant gait problem, testing the patient's gait inside the examination room (or simply observing the patient when he or she walks into or out of the room) may suffice to prove that gait is normal. When an abnormality of gait is suspected, watching the gait for a longer distance, such as in a hallway, may be necessary.
2. Ask the patient to walk, and observe the patient's base (how far the legs are apart), stride, and balance. In some cases, you may only need to see

the patient walk a few steps to confirm that the gait is normal, and, in other cases, you may want to watch the patient walk a longer distance.

3. Ask the patient to turn around and walk back to the starting point. Watch how the patient turns (this is particularly important in the assessment of parkinsonism; see Chapter 46, Examination of the Patient with a Movement Disorder), and then observe the gait again as the patient walks back.

Tandem Gait

1. Ask the patient to walk a straight line, "like walking a tightrope." It is often helpful to show the patient a line on the floor on which to walk.
2. Observe the patient's ability to walk a few (e.g., four or five) steps in this way.

Walking on the Heels or Toes

1. To test heel walking, ask the patient to walk forward on his or her heels (dorsiflexing the feet). Observe as the patient walks four or five steps forward.
2. To test toe walking, ask the patient to walk forward on his or her toes (plantar flexing the feet), and observe as the patient walks four or five steps forward.

NORMAL FINDINGS

The normal gait should have a narrow base (the feet should be approximately shoulder-width apart), and it should be steady with good stride length. Patients should be able to perform tandem gait without significant difficulty and without needing to hold on to the wall or falling to either side. It is not unusual for elderly patients to have some difficulty with tandem gait, however; if the gait is otherwise normal, mild problems with tandem gait can probably be considered a variation of normal in this population.

If tested, patients should also be able to walk a few steps on their heels (maintaining dorsiflexion of the feet) and their toes (maintaining plantar flexion of the feet) without difficulty.

ABNORMAL FINDINGS

Routine Gait Testing

- A wide-based and unsteady gait, resembling the gait that can be seen from alcohol intoxication (a drunken gait), is called *gait ataxia* and suggests cerebellar dysfunction. If the patient with an ataxic gait does not have a propensity to fall toward one particular side, the pathology is most likely in the midline (vermis) of the cerebellum. An ataxic gait with consistent veering to one side suggests dysfunction of the cerebellar hemisphere on the side that the patient is falling toward (i.e., falling toward the left suggests left cerebellar dysfunction).

- A wide-based, unsteady (ataxic) gait can also be seen due to severe sensory dysfunction in the feet and legs; this is referred to as a *sensory ataxia*. Sensory ataxias predominantly occur when there is severe proprioceptive and vibratory sensation loss in the lower extremities.

- A narrow-based shuffling gait, often with a stooped posture, is called a *parkinsonian gait*. There may be diminished arm swing, difficulty making turns without taking extra steps, and a resting tremor of the hands, depending on the cause and severity of the underlying dysfunction. The finding of a parkinsonian gait suggests Parkinson's disease or other causes of parkinsonism (see Chapter 46, Examination of the Patient with a Movement Disorder).

- Some patients have difficulty initiating steps after standing and may even complain that their feet are "glued" to the floor; after initiating gait, their steps are short and hesitant. This gait is called an *apractic gait* because the patient has normal motor mechanisms, but the brain can't figure out how to perform the sequence of maneuvers to walk (*apraxia* refers to the inability to perform a complex task despite normal motor function). The finding of an apractic gait suggests frontal lobe dysfunction, such as can occur from some chronic dementing illnesses, hydrocephalus, or structural frontal lobe lesions.
- Patients with a hemiparesis often have a characteristic hemiparetic gait. The leg is stiff and extended with circumduction at the hip; the affected arm is also usually held in a flexed position. Hemiparetic gaits usually occur from unilateral cerebral hemispheric lesions affecting the corticospinal tracts; these usually cause upper motor neuron weakness predominantly affecting extensors of the arm and flexors of the leg, with relative preservation of strength in arm flexors and leg extensors.
- Patients with bilateral upper motor neuron weakness in the legs have bilaterally stiff legs, which, because of the bilateral circumduction, have a scissoring quality as the patient propels forward. This paraparetic gait disorder most commonly occurs due to spinal cord dysfunction, but it can also be seen due to bilateral cerebral hemisphere lesions.
- Weakness in foot dorsiflexion (foot drop) causes a characteristic gait called a *steppage gait*; the patient needs to lift the leg to avoid tripping on the involved foot. This gait disorder, which can be unilateral or bilateral, can occur due to any cause of foot dorsiflexion weakness, usually from peripheral etiologies.
- Another kind of gait abnormality that can occur due to nonneurologic causes is called an *antalgic gait*. This refers to the gait that occurs due to pain, particularly pain in an extremity, such as due to a hip problem or other musculoskeletal process.

Tandem Gait Testing

Abnormalities on tandem gait manifest as unsteadiness during the maneuver or inability to perform tandem gait without the likelihood of falling. Although most likely to be affected due to cerebellar dysfunction, difficulties with tandem gait are nonspecific and can occur due to any of the gait disorders described previously.

Heel or Toe Walking

- Difficulty walking forward on one or both heels suggests any cause of unilateral or bilateral foot dorsiflexion weakness.
- Difficulty walking forward on the one or both toes suggests any cause of unilateral or bilateral foot plantar-flexion weakness. The finding of difficulty walking on the plantar-flexed foot can be a particularly helpful sign when weakness of plantar flexion is suspected but not seen on routine motor testing. This is because power in plantar flexors is usually quite strong, and it may take the patient's inability to lift his or her own weight to confirm weakness of plantar flexion.

ADDITIONAL POINTS

- It is sometimes difficult to distinguish a parkinsonian gait from an apractic gait. Parkinsonian gaits are usually more narrow based than the gaits that occur due to frontal lobe dysfunction, however. Apractic gaits are sometimes referred to as *magnetic gaits* because the feet appear stuck to the floor.

- Tandem gait can sometimes be improved by asking the patient to walk quickly. In patients who are cautious and deliberate and seem slightly unsteady when performing this maneuver, you may find them to be more steady (i.e., normal) as they speed up.
- Although this chapter discusses the evaluation of gait for diagnostic purposes, another important purpose of gait evaluation is to assess the patient's safety in ambulation.

Chapter 40

PERFORMING A COMPLETE NEUROLOGIC EXAMINATION

PURPOSE OF THE COMPLETE NEUROLOGIC EXAMINATION

The purpose of performing a complete neurologic examination is to look for clues to the localization and mechanism of your patient's neurologic disease process.

WHEN TO PERFORM THE COMPLETE NEUROLOGIC EXAMINATION

A complete neurologic examination should be performed on all patients who present with symptoms that may be due to neurologic dysfunction, such as disorders of consciousness or cognition, dizziness, headache, vision, muscle strength or movement, sensory function, gait, or balance. The neurologic examination should always be performed after a neurologic history has been obtained.

As described in the preceding chapters, there are basic examination elements that should be performed on all patients and basic elements that can be omitted in some situations. For example, pin sensation should be tested on patients who have a sensory complaint, but it can reasonably be omitted in many patients who don't. There are also procedures that only need to be performed in specific clinical situations, such as oculocephalic testing in the comatose patient, the Dix-Hallpike maneuver in patients with possible positional vertigo, or testing for meningismus in patients with acute headache; such clinical scenario–specific neurologic examination procedures are discussed in Section 3, Neurologic Examination in Common Clinical Scenarios.

NEUROANATOMY OF THE COMPLETE NEUROLOGIC EXAMINATION

The basic relevant neuroanatomy underlying each examination element is briefly described in the previous chapters.

EQUIPMENT NEEDED TO PERFORM THE COMPLETE NEUROLOGIC EXAMINATION

The items needed to perform the complete neurologic examination are listed in Chapter 1, Role of the Neurologic History and Examination in Neurologic Diagnosis.

HOW TO PERFORM THE COMPLETE NEUROLOGIC EXAMINATION

The following, in the order shown, is one step-by-step method of performing the complete neurologic examination in a typical patient (elements of the examination that are optional depending on the clinical situation are listed in parentheses):

Examine the Mental Status

1. If any dysfunction of alertness, language, memory, or any other aspect of cognitive function is suspected or is a concern, or if an abnormality is suggested during your history-taking, formally test mental status as discussed in Chapters 5 through 8; otherwise, informally assess mental status while taking the history and proceed to the examination of the cranial nerves.

Examine the Cranial Nerves

2. Look at the resting size and symmetry of the pupils (see Chapter 10, Examination of the Pupils).
3. Examine the response of each pupil to light (see Chapter 10, Examination of the Pupils).
4. (If indicated, test the pupillary response to near or test for an afferent pupillary defect, as described in Chapter 10, Examination of the Pupils.)
5. Perform a funduscopic examination to look at the optic discs (see Chapter 11, Funduscopic Examination).
6. (If indicated, assess visual acuity, as described in Chapter 12, Examination of Visual Acuity.)
7. Test visual fields to confrontation (see Chapter 13, Visual Field Examination).
8. Test eye movements: first test horizontal eye movements, then test vertical eye movements (see Chapter 14, Examination of Eye Movements).
9. (If indicated, test facial sensation, as described in Chapter 15, Examination of Facial Sensation.)
10. Test facial strength (see Chapter 16, Examination of Facial Strength).
11. (If indicated, check jaw strength, as described in Chapter 17, Examination of Jaw Strength.)
12. (If indicated, check hearing and air and bone conduction, as described in Chapter 18, Examination of Hearing.)
13. Look at palatal elevation to phonation (see Chapter 19, Examination of Palatal Function).
14. Assess that the protruded tongue is midline and that it can wiggle from side-to-side (see Chapter 20, Examination of Tongue Movement).
15. (If indicated, as described in Chapter 21, Examination of the Sterno-cleidomastoid and Trapezius Muscles, check the strength of the sterno-cleidomastoid and trapezius muscles.)
16. (If indicated, examine taste, as described in Chapter 22, Examination of Taste.)
17. (If indicated, examine the patient's sense of smell, as described in Chapter 23, Examination of Smell.)

Examine Motor Function

18. Test for drift of the outstretched arms (see Chapter 25, Examination of Upper Extremity Muscle Strength).
19. Look for fasciculations or atrophy in the muscles (see Chapter 24, Approach to the Motor Examination).

20. Test upper extremity muscle strength (see Chapter 25, Examination of Upper Extremity Muscle Strength). The following are muscles that can be quickly and easily tested in all patients as a good sampling of proximal and distal muscles in multiple root and nerve distributions:
    - Deltoid
    - Biceps
    - Triceps
    - Wrist extensors
    - Finger extensors
    - Interossei

    Additional upper extremity muscles, as described in Chapter 25, Examination of Upper Extremity Muscle Strength, may need to be tested when weakness is found or you are trying to pinpoint a particular nerve or root distribution of weakness.

21. Test lower extremity muscle strength (see Chapter 26, Examination of Lower Extremity Muscle Strength). The following can be quickly and easily tested in all patients as a good sampling of proximal and distal muscles in multiple root and nerve distributions:
    - Hip flexors
    - Extension at the knees
    - Flexion at the knees
    - Foot dorsiflexion
    - Foot plantar flexion

    Additional lower extremity muscles, as described in Chapter 26, Examination of Lower Extremity Muscle Strength, may need to be tested when weakness is found or you are trying to pinpoint a particular nerve or root distribution of weakness.

22. (If indicated, assess tone, as described in Chapter 27, Examination of Tone.)

Examine Sensory Function

23. Test vibration sense (and position sense, if indicated), as described in Chapter 30, Examination of Vibration and Position Sensation.
24. (If indicated, examine pinprick sensation, as discussed in Chapter 29, Examination of Pinprick Sensation.)
25. (If indicated, examine cortical sensation, as described in Chapter 31, Examination of Cortical Sensation.)

Examine Cerebellar Function

26. Test the finger-to-nose maneuver (see Chapter 34, Testing of Upper Extremity Cerebellar Function).
27. (If indicated, test the heel-to-shin maneuver, as described in Chapter 35, Testing of Lower Extremity Cerebellar Function.)

Examine the Muscle Stretch Reflexes

28. Test the biceps jerks, triceps jerks, knee jerks, and ankle jerks (see Chapter 37, Examination of the Muscle Stretch Reflexes).

Examine for the Babinski Response

29. Test for the Babinski response on each foot (see Chapter 38, Testing for the Babinski Response).

Examine the Gait and Test for the Romberg Sign

30. Watch the patient walk (see Chapter 39, Examination of Gait.)

31. Watch the patient perform a tandem gait (see Chapter 39, Examination of Gait).
32. (If indicated, watch the patient walk forward on his or her heels and then on his or her toes, as described in Chapter 39, Examination of Gait.)
33. Test for the Romberg sign (see Chapter 32, Romberg Testing).

NORMAL FINDINGS

Normal findings for each component of the neurologic examination are discussed in previous chapters.

ABNORMAL FINDINGS

Abnormal findings for each component of the neurologic examination are discussed in previous chapters.

ADDITIONAL POINTS

- The items listed in How to Perform the Complete Neurologic Examination (even excluding the examination elements in parentheses) constitute a thorough neurologic examination. With practice, this examination can be performed quickly and easily, and it can give you a good idea of the integrity of your patient's central and peripheral nervous system; any abnormalities you find should help you in localizing your patient's neurologic dysfunction.
- There is no single correct order or way to perform a neurologic examination. The method described in How to Perform the Complete Neurologic Examination, starting with the mental status, then proceeding down from the head (cranial nerves) and ending with the toes (the Babinski sign) and gait, is one common method. Choose an order that you are comfortable with and try to be consistent to avoid forgetting important examination elements. It's usually a good idea to do all of the examination elements of a category together (e.g., perform all muscle strength testing together as one component of the examination, starting with the upper extremities and proceeding to the lower extremities).

Neurologic Examination in Common Clinical Scenarios

Chapter 41

TAILORING THE NEUROLOGIC HISTORY AND EXAMINATION TO THE CLINICAL SCENARIO

GOAL

The goal of tailoring the history and examination to the clinical scenario is to obtain the information that's needed to help figure out what's wrong with your patient.

PATHOPHYSIOLOGY

In each of the following chapters of this section, the basic relevant pathophysiology underlying various common symptoms or syndromes is discussed as a background to the appropriate historical and examination procedures and findings helpful in diagnosis.

TAILORING THE HISTORY TO THE CLINICAL SCENARIO

Although a thorough neurologic history should be attempted in all patients, there are pieces of information that are of particular interest in some clinical scenarios more than others. These discriminating historical features are reviewed throughout the chapters that follow.

HOW TO TAILOR THE EXAMINATION TO THE CLINICAL SCENARIO

- In all patients with neurologic symptoms, an appropriately thorough neurologic examination should be attempted, as discussed in Chapter 40, Performing a Complete Neurologic Examination. Depending on the clinical scenario, however, some examination elements are likely to be more helpful than others in getting you to the diagnosis, and you should concentrate particularly on these during the examination. For example, in a patient who presents with diplopia, the examination of eye movements is most likely to be the most telling examination procedure diagnostically. In the following chapters, the importance of specific examination procedures and findings in various common clinical syndromes is discussed.
- There are clinical situations in which the neurologic examination is necessarily limited, often because of the neurologic symptoms themselves, such as the acutely confused patient or the comatose patient; in situations such as these, important diagnostic information can be learned if you

know what clues are most important and how they should be found. These examination findings are discussed in the relevant chapters that follow.

- Certain examination procedures can be helpful in specific clinical settings but are unnecessary at other times. Examples include oculocephalic testing in coma, the Dix-Hallpike maneuver in patients with positional vertigo, and testing for meningismus in patients with acute headache; syndrome-specific tests such as these are discussed in the relevant chapters of this section.

Chapter 42

EXAMINATION OF THE COMATOSE PATIENT

GOAL

The goal of the history and examination of the comatose patient is to look for clues to the localization and etiology of the process causing coma.

PATHOPHYSIOLOGY OF COMA

Normal consciousness depends on the cerebral hemispheres to provide cognition and the reticular formation of the upper brainstem (from the mid-pons and above) to provide alertness. Coma, the absence of consciousness, can occur only due to dysfunction of both cerebral hemispheres, dysfunction of the upper brainstem, or a combination of bilateral hemisphere and upper brainstem dysfunction.

Much of the examination of the comatose patient focuses on assessing brainstem function. This is because most structural brainstem processes causing coma produce easily identified abnormalities on examination, but structural disorders of the hemispheres or diffuse metabolic disorders generally show preservation of brainstem function on examination. Therefore, if the brainstem is functioning normally, a structural brainstem process (such as a brainstem stroke or brainstem compression) is unlikely to be the cause of coma; the process causing coma would then most likely be due to structural lesions affecting both of the hemispheres or a diffuse metabolic process.

TAKING THE HISTORY OF A COMATOSE PATIENT

The history needs to be obtained from witnesses, family, or friends for any clues they may provide to the cause of the patient's problem. If possible, try to obtain information regarding the temporal course of development of impaired consciousness, any recent systemic or neurologic symptoms, head trauma, the patient's past medical and social history, medications, and any other potentially relevant available historical information.

HOW TO EXAMINE THE COMATOSE PATIENT

General Examination

As part of a detailed general and neurologic examination, look in the fundi for evidence of papilledema (see Fig. 11–2), which would suggest increased intracranial pressure, or retinal hemorrhages (see Fig. 11–3), which would suggest subarachnoid hemorrhage. Look for evidence for a basilar skull fracture by looking in the ear canals for blood, inspecting the mastoid areas for ecchymosis (Battle's sign), or finding ecchymosis around the eyes (raccoon eyes). Fever suggests the possibility of meningitis, encephalitis, or sepsis. Meningismus (see Chapter 45, Examination of the Patient with Headache) is a clue to meningitis or subarachnoid hemorrhage but may be an insensitive sign in deep unconsciousness.

Assess the Level of Consciousness

Assess the patient's level of consciousness within the continuum from drowsiness to coma by looking at the response to external stimuli, as follows:

- Assess response to verbal stimuli by calling the patient's name loudly or asking the patient to follow a simple command, such as "open your eyes," "blink your eyes," or "stick out your tongue."
- Assess response to visual stimuli first by opening the patient's eyes and seeing if the patient attends to you. Test the patient's response to visual threat by holding the patient's eyes open and assess whether the patient blinks when you make a quick motion with your hands in front of each eye. To avoid inadvertently producing a corneal reflex from air pushed into the cornea, bring your hands in from the sides when testing visual threat.
- In any potentially comatose patient, ensure that the patient does not actually have the *locked-in syndrome* by holding the patient's eyes open and asking the patient to look down. Patients with the locked-in syndrome are not comatose. They are awake but quadriplegic and have paralysis of horizontal eye movements; they can communicate only by looking down or blinking on command. This syndrome occurs due to large lesions of the base of the pons, usually infarction.

Assess Resting Eye Position

Open the patient's eyes and look at the resting position of the eyes for any tonic (persistent) deviation of the eyes to one side (called a *gaze preference*), as follows:

- A gaze preference away from the side of a hemiparesis is consistent with a large acute cerebral hemispheric lesion. This is because the frontal eye fields (see Chapter 14, Examination of Eye Movements) of each hemisphere move the eyes to the contralateral side; therefore, a large lesion of one of the hemispheres causes the eyes to deviate toward the damaged hemisphere because of the unopposed action of the intact frontal eye field from the opposite healthy hemisphere. *In other words, the eyes look to the side of an acute hemispheric lesion and away from the hemiparesis.*
- A gaze preference toward the side of a hemiparesis is consistent with an acute lesion in the brainstem, particularly the pons. This is because the lateral gaze mechanisms located on each side of the pons move the eyes to the ipsilateral side; therefore, a lesion of one side of the pons causes the eyes to deviate away from the damaged side of the brainstem because of the unopposed action of the intact lateral gaze center on the opposite healthy side of the pons. *In other words, the eyes look away from the side of a pontine lesion and toward the hemiparesis.*
- Sustained downgaze deviation of both eyes can be seen in the setting of processes that affect the posterior (dorsal) upper midbrain/thalamic region, such as pineal tumors.

Observe for Any Spontaneous Eye Movements

Open the patient's eyes and look for any spontaneous eye movements, as follows:

- Roving eye movements are slow conjugate horizontal movements of the eyes from one side to the other. The presence of spontaneous roving eye movements implies that the brainstem mechanisms in the pons and midbrain that move each eye laterally and medially, respectively, are intact. Roving eye movements are seen in situations in which there is bilateral hemispheric dysfunction with relative preservation of brainstem function, such as anoxic encephalopathies.

- Ocular bobbing consists of downward jerks of both eyes, which then slowly return upward to mid-position before jerking downward again. Ocular bobbing is seen in patients who have lost their horizontal gaze mechanisms due to a lesion of the base of the pons, but who have preservation of the mechanisms that control downward vertical gaze in the midbrain. Because ocular bobbing is seen in patients with pontine lesions, these patients should particularly be assessed for the locked-in state.

Assess Reflex Eye Movements

Testing of reflex horizontal eye movements is important when trying to decide if brainstem function is intact, but you haven't observed any spontaneous eye movements. You don't need to test reflex eye movements when spontaneous horizontal roving eye movements are seen, because their presence already tells you that the brainstem control of eye movements is intact. Test reflex eye movements as follows:

- Test for the oculocephalic (doll's eyes) reflex by turning the patient's head to one side and then to the other. In a comatose patient whose brainstem is intact, turning the head to one side should result in conjugate deviation of both eyes to the contralateral side. In other words, turning the head to the left should result in deviation of both eyes to the right, and turning the head to the right should result in deviation of both eyes to the left. This can be reported as a "positive" or "intact" doll's eyes response, or to be even clearer, can be reported as "turning the head resulted in bilateral conjugate horizontal eye deviation to the opposite side."
- Test the oculovestibular (cold caloric) reflex if the oculocephalic (doll's eyes) maneuver fails to show normal horizontal eye movements or cannot be performed. This test is most important clinically in the assessment of possible brain death (see Brain Death section). Oculocephalic testing does not need to be performed if normal horizontal eye movements have already been observed spontaneously or during the doll's eyes maneuver, because normal brainstem control of eye movements has already been proven. To perform cold caloric testing:
  1. Raise the patient's head (or the head of the bed) up to approximately 30 degrees.
  2. Using an otoscope, look to be sure that the external auditory canals are patent and that the tympanic membranes are intact.
  3. Prepare a mixture of ice water and draw the ice-cold water up into a large syringe. Attach a large-gauge plastic intravenous catheter (with the needle removed) to the end of the syringe.
  4. Place the catheter within one of the ear canals (don't go too deep to avoid piercing the tympanic membrane). Slowly instill up to 100 mL of the ice-cold water into the ear canal.
  5. Observe the response of the eyes for the next 1 to 2 minutes.
  6. After waiting at least 5 minutes, perform the same maneuver on the other side.
- In a comatose patient whose brainstem is intact, instilling ice water into the ear canal should result in conjugate deviation of both eyes toward the side of the irrigated ear. In other words, instilling ice water into the left ear should result in deviation of both eyes to the left, and instilling ice water into the right ear should result in deviation of both eyes to the right. This can be reported as a "positive" or "intact" caloric response, or to be even clearer, can be specifically reported as "cold caloric irrigation of each ear resulted in bilateral conjugate horizontal eye deviation to the side of the irrigated ear."

- The presence of intact horizontal eye movements spontaneously or on oculocephalic or oculovestibular testing implies that the brainstem is structurally intact, and the coma is most likely due to structural lesions affecting both of the hemispheres or a diffuse metabolic process affecting the hemispheres or brainstem.

Assess Pupillary Function

Assess resting pupillary size and pupillary responses to light for diagnostic clues, as follows:

- Bilateral pinpoint (1 mm) pupils suggest a pontine lesion, such as infarction or hemorrhage. On close inspection, these pupils do constrict to light.
- Bilateral mid-position (4 to 6 mm) pupils that are unreactive to light can be seen due to midbrain lesions.
- A unilaterally dilated pupil, regardless of whether there are other motor signs of third nerve dysfunction, such as lateral and downward deviation of the eye, suggests a third nerve palsy (see Chapter 10, Examination of the Pupils, and Chapter 14, Examination of Eye Movements). In the comatose patient, this suggests herniation of a unilateral hemispheric mass lesion causing pressure on the third nerve or its nucleus in the midbrain. A third nerve palsy can also be seen from other compressive lesions, such as a posterior communicating artery aneurysm.
- Metabolic disorders generally don't affect the pupils, except for opiate intoxication, which leads to small pupils that react to light, and anticholinergic drugs, such as atropine, that may cause dilated and unreactive pupils.

Assess Motor Function

Observe the patient for spontaneous movements of the extremities and the presence of abnormal posturing (which may be seen spontaneously or after noxious stimuli), as follows:

- Diminished movement of the extremities on one side of the body compared to the other suggests a hemiparesis. A hemiparesis can also be suspected by observing that one of the legs is externally rotated.
- Decerebrate (extensor) posturing is characterized by extension of the arms with extension of the legs. There may also be extension of the neck. Although posturing is not entirely specific in terms of localization, the presence of extensor posturing generally suggests severe midbrain or pontine dysfunction, which may be due to intrinsic brainstem lesions or compression from a hemispheric mass. Extensor posturing can also rarely be seen in severe metabolic encephalopathies.
- Decorticate (flexor) posturing is characterized by flexion of the arms with extension of the legs. The presence of flexor posturing generally suggests higher (e.g., hemispheric) dysfunction than extensor posturing.
- If necessary, assess the patient's motor response to noxious stimuli, such as pressing on the nail bed. This may result in reflex motor patterns consistent with decorticate or decerebrate posturing, which may not have been otherwise evident spontaneously, or it may result in a more voluntary type of withdrawal. Although it may be difficult to distinguish voluntary withdrawal from a purely reflex response, abduction of the shoulder or hip is likely to be a higher level response.

Assess Breathing Patterns

Most comatose patients are likely to be mechanically ventilated when you examine them, so the interpretation of breathing patterns is usually not a significant part of the diagnostic process. There are some patterns you should be aware of, however, including the following:

- *Cheyne-Stokes respirations* are characterized by increasing and decreasing amplitudes of respiration with intervening apneic periods. Cheyne-Stokes respirations are typically seen due to bilateral hemispheric or bilateral thalamic dysfunction, including dysfunction from hypoxia and other metabolic disorders.
- Central neurogenic hyperventilation is an uncommon respiratory pattern diagnosed by the presence of sustained hyperventilation in the absence of hypoxia or other metabolic causes of hyperventilation. Central neurogenic hyperventilation has been associated with midbrain or pontine lesions.

Brain Death

The details of the clinical assessment of brain death are beyond the scope of this text, but some points are summarized here. Brain death is the irreversible absence of all function of the brain due to a catastrophic process involving the entirety of both cerebral hemispheres and the brainstem. In addition to confirming complete unresponsiveness, much of the clinical assessment of brain death focuses on confirming the absence of all brainstem function, including the following findings on bedside testing of brainstem function:

- Absent pupillary responses to light.
- Absent eye movements, including absent eye movements to oculovestibular (caloric) testing bilaterally.
- Absent corneal reflexes. To test corneal reflexes, lightly touch the cornea of one of the patient's eyes with a cotton swab. The normal response in the patient with an intact brainstem is to blink both eyes; the absence of any blink to this maneuver is abnormal. Repeat by touching the other cornea with the cotton swab.
- Absent gag reflex and absent cough to tracheal suctioning.
- No motor responses, including absent spontaneous movements and the absence of any kind of posturing (decerebrate or decorticate) to noxious stimuli. Muscle stretch reflexes and Babinski signs, however, may be present, because these are spinal cord reflexes.
- The absence of breathing and respiratory drive. This requires performing an apnea test* to confirm the absence of any respiratory drive to hypercarbia at least 20 mm Hg above the baseline PCO_2 level.

ADDITIONAL COMMENTS

There is often confusion about the purpose of caloric testing in coma (some think it is a test for nystagmus). In clinical neurology, caloric testing is performed only in coma, with the specific intention of looking for evidence of brainstem function by observing for (normal) conjugate eye deviation toward the ear that has been infused with cold water. Nystagmus is not an expected finding when caloric testing is performed in coma. On the other hand, if caloric testing were performed on a patient who was awake (which we don't intend to do), nystagmus would occur, with the fast phase away from the irrigated ear; this nystagmus would represent an attempt by the brain to compensate for the slow deviation of the eyes toward the irrigated ear.

---

*For further details about the determination of brain death and the performance of apnea testing, see Wijdicks EF. The diagnosis of brain death. *N Engl J Med* 2001;344:1215–1221.

Chapter 43

EXAMINATION OF THE PATIENT WITH ALTERED MENTAL STATUS

GOAL

The main goal of the history and examination of the patient with an alteration in mental status is to look for evidence of whether the patient's symptoms represent a diffuse encephalopathic process, a dementing illness, or a symptom of focal brain dysfunction.

PATHOPHYSIOLOGY OF ALTERED MENTAL STATUS

Mental status can be affected by disorders that affect the level of consciousness (alertness) or disorders that affect cognitive function (see Chapter 5, Approach to the Mental Status Examination).

Disorders of Level of Consciousness

The pathophysiology of changes in consciousness severe enough to cause coma are discussed in Chapter 42, Examination of the Comatose Patient. All of the same processes and mechanisms, either focal or diffuse, that can cause coma can also present as lesser degrees of altered consciousness. One common cause of disordered consciousness, manifested as an acute confusional state, is a *toxic-metabolic encephalopathy*, the neurologists' term for delirium; this represents the severe altered mental status that can occur in the setting of a systemic illness or as a result of many metabolic or toxic disorders.

Disorders of Cognition

Dementias are neurologic illnesses that impair function in memory and at least one other aspect of cognitive function, such as judgment, personality, visual-spatial ability, language, and abstract thinking. Causes of dementia include, among others, degenerative illnesses (e.g., Alzheimer's disease, frontotemporal dementia, and Lewy body dementia), multiinfarct dementia, and Creutzfeldt-Jakob disease. Dementing illnesses, for the most part, affect cognitive function without impairing the level of consciousness. Cognitive function can also be affected by any focal neurologic process affecting cognitively important cortical regions.

TAKING THE HISTORY OF A PATIENT WITH AN ALTERED MENTAL STATUS

Depending on the severity of the illness, patients with an alteration in consciousness or cognition may or may not be able to provide much history or have insight into their dysfunction. In most cases, details of the history need to be obtained from family members (see Chapter 42, Examination of the Comatose Patient).

- Ask about the time course of the change in mental status. An acute onset of altered mental status over seconds suggests an acute focal process, such as stroke affecting cognitive regions. A subacute onset over hours or days would be expected in most toxic-metabolic encephalopathies or many structural processes. A chronic and progressive course over months or years would be expected in dementing illnesses (although Creutzfeldt-Jakob disease would be more rapid, and vascular dementia should have a step-wise course).

- Ask about the details of the dysfunction. Lethargy or agitation (or both) would be expected in delirium; hallucinations (especially visual) may also be present. Patients with dementias usually present with recent memory impairment as their most prominent symptom or may have personality and behavioral changes, but they rarely have impairment in their level of consciousness, at least not early in their course.
- Ask about the presence of new systemic symptoms that would suggest toxic-metabolic dysfunction in the acutely confused patient or focal neurologic symptoms that might suggest a focal process.
- Look for any medications the patient may be taking that might be causing central nervous system side effects.
- Ask about symptoms of depression, such as changes in mood, appetite, and sleep, that might suggest the presence of a pseudodementia.

HOW TO EXAMINE THE PATIENT WITH ALTERED MENTAL STATUS

- In the patient with acutely or subacutely altered mental status, approach your general assessment as described in Chapter 42, Examination of the Comatose Patient. Fever would suggest the possibility of meningitis, encephalitis, or sepsis (systemic infection is a common cause of toxic-metabolic encephalopathy).
- Assess the patient's level of consciousness by observation. In the absence of other significant focal neurologic signs (see below), any impairment in alertness suggests the possibility of a diffuse (toxic-metabolic) encephalopathic process.
- Chapters 5, 6, and 7 describe the details of the mental status examination, which should be attempted in all patients with any alteration in mental status. In particular, assess the patient's orientation, language, concentration, and memory.
- In the patient with an acute onset of confusion, always consider the possibility that the patient might have Wernicke's aphasia (see Chapter 6, Language Testing); listen carefully for any paraphasic errors and neologisms.
- In those patients in whom a detailed motor and sensory examination may not be possible because of confusion, look for gross asymmetries in motor function, including testing for drift, to assess for evidence of focal brain dysfunction. Also, look for obvious reflex asymmetry or a Babinski sign.
- A helpful examination finding in many patients with toxic-metabolic encephalopathies is asterixis. Asterixis consists of brief, often subtle, downward flapping or jerking of the extended hands due to lapses in muscle tone. Asterixis is seen in many toxic-metabolic encephalopathic processes but is particularly common in hepatic and uremic encephalopathies. Perform the following to test for asterixis:
  1. Ask your patient to hold his or her arms extended, directly in front of him or her.
  2. Have the patient dorsiflex his or her wrists so that the hands are straight up, "like you are stopping traffic."
  3. Observe the patient for at least a few seconds as he or she tries to maintain the hands in this position. Look for any subtle lapses in tone (asterixis), manifested as brief downward jerks of the hands at the wrists.

- In some patients with severe toxic-metabolic encephalopathies, especially those of hepatic or uremic origin, diffuse myoclonus (see Chapter 46, Examination of the Patient with a Movement Disorder) may also be observed and can be a prominent clinical finding. Myoclonic jerks of the extremities can also be seen in Creutzfeldt-Jakob disease.

- In patients with dementia, the Folstein Mini-Mental State Examination (MMSE), a standardized battery of various cognitive tasks, is often used to assess global cognitive function (see Chapter 5, Approach to the Mental Status Examination); the MMSE score can be followed serially over subsequent visits to assess for change in the patient's cognition as an adjunct to the interval history. Another advantage of using the MMSE is that it allows you to remember to test most of the important cognitive tasks (always report each incorrect item and not just the absolute score out of the total of 30 points). Although the score on the MMSE correlates with severity of cognitive dysfunction, the absolute score is not diagnostic of any particular cause of dementia or any other cause of encephalopathy.

- Gait examination can provide clues to the cause of dementing illnesses. A parkinsonian gait (see Chapter 39, Examination of Gait) would suggest the possibility of Lewy body dementia. Gait disorders, however, particularly apraxia of gait (described in Chapter 39, Examination of Gait), may be seen late in the course of any severe chronic dementia as a sign of frontal lobe dysfunction. Patients with the syndrome of normal pressure hydrocephalus would be particularly likely to manifest an apraxia of gait as an early finding.

- Gegenhalten rigidity (described in Chapter 27, Examination of Tone) can be seen late in the course of any severe chronic dementia, but it is a nonspecific sign. Other classic frontal release signs, such as the glabellar reflex (continual blinking when the patient's mid-forehead is repeatedly tapped), the grasp reflex (flexion of the patient's fingers and grasping of the patient's hand when lightly brushed by the examiner's hand), and the palmomental reflex (twitch of the patient's ipsilateral chin when the patient's palm is lightly scratched by a blunt object) are also nonspecific, are of doubtful efficacy in neurologic assessment of any patient, and can be skipped.

Chapter 44

EXAMINATION OF THE DIZZY PATIENT

GOAL

The main goal of the history and examination of the patient with dizziness is to determine whether the patient's dizziness is actually due to lightheadedness, imbalance, or vertigo, paving the way for the most appropriate further investigation and treatment.

PATHOPHYSIOLOGY OF DIZZINESS

Patients may use the word *dizzy* to describe several different symptoms, including a sensation of lightheadedness, imbalance, or movement (vertigo).

- *Lightheadedness* implies a sensation of impending loss of consciousness, also called *presyncope*. Episodic lightheadedness suggests episodes of global cerebral hypoperfusion, such as from cardiac causes or orthostatic hypotension.
- *Imbalance* is a sensation of gait instability (disequilibrium) that may range from subtle to severe. Patients may especially interpret their imbalance as "dizziness" when their gait dysfunction is subtle, because they may be unaware that their feeling is really an imbalanced sensation.
- *Vertigo* refers to an illusory sensation of motion. Most patients with vertigo describe a feeling of rotation of the environment or in their head, but vertigo can also include any feeling of movement, such as a feeling of tilting or swaying. Vertigo occurs due to disorders of the vestibular system, either peripheral (the inner ear or the vestibular nerve) or central (brainstem or cerebellum).

TAKING THE HISTORY OF A DIZZY PATIENT

When evaluating a patient with a complaint of dizziness, the main goal of the history is to try to determine what the patient means by "dizzy." The first step is to simply ask the patient, "What do you mean by dizzy?" Let the patient tell you, in his or her own words, what he or she means, and try to avoid putting words in the patient's mouth. Additional clues to the cause of dizziness that can be gleaned by the history alone are listed below.

Lightheadedness

- Patients with lightheadedness (presyncope) usually can describe their feeling as that of "lightheadedness" or a feeling "like I might pass out." A history of any of the episodes progressing to true loss of consciousness is further evidence that the patient's symptoms fit into this category of dizziness.
- Ask about any associated cardiac symptoms, such as palpitations or chest pain, although the absence of these symptoms does not exclude a cardiac cause.
- Lightheadedness occurring only after standing suggests orthostatic hypotension.

Imbalance

- Patients with imbalance as the cause of their dizziness usually can describe their feeling as something like an "off-balanced" or "unsteady" sensation, and they should be symptomatic when standing or walking but not when lying or sitting.
- The historical finding of worsened imbalance when standing in the dark (e.g., walking to the bathroom at night) or with eyes closed (e.g., in the shower) suggests proprioceptive dysfunction. Even in the absence of a positive Romberg test, these historical clues are strongly suggestive of proprioceptive problems, such as can occur due to peripheral neuropathies or spinal cord (posterior column) problems.

Vertigo

- Patients with vertigo usually can describe their feeling as that of a spinning, moving, or tilting sensation.
- Ask about any associated brainstem symptoms, such as double vision, or numbness or weakness of the face or of the extremities. The presence of brainstem symptoms in patients with vertigo is strongly suggestive of brainstem dysfunction (e.g., ischemia) as the cause; their absence, however, doesn't exclude the possibility of a central (brainstem or cerebellar) cause of vertigo.
- Hearing complaints, such as unilateral hearing loss or tinnitus, occurring in association with vertigo suggest a peripheral labyrinthine disorder.
- Paroxysmal vertigo brought on by changes in head position, such as when turning, bending over, or rolling over in bed, is highly suggestive of the clinical syndrome of benign paroxysmal positional vertigo (BPPV), which occurs due to the presence of calcium carbonate crystals floating in one of the semicircular canals.
- Nausea and vomiting is a nonspecific accompaniment of vertigo and can occur with vertigo of peripheral or central etiologies.

HOW TO EXAMINE THE DIZZY PATIENT

After obtaining the history, you should hopefully have a pretty good idea whether your patient's dizziness is due to lightheadedness, imbalance, or vertigo. The examination is then performed to find evidence to support or refute your hypothesis and provide further information regarding possible etiologies. Listed below are specific examination elements, depending on your clinical suspicion, that can be helpful.

Lightheadedness

- In the patient with episodic lightheadedness, be certain (as in any new patient visit) to obtain your patient's blood pressure and pulse, and also perform a bedside cardiac examination.
- Check lying and standing blood pressure in any patient whose symptoms suggest the possibility of orthostatic hypotension:
  1. Have the patient lie flat in bed for a few minutes, then check the patient's supine blood pressure and pulse.
  2. Ask the patient to stand. (It's usually not necessary to check a sitting blood pressure and pulse, unless the patient can't tolerate the standing position.)
  3. After the patient has been upright for approximately 2 to 3 minutes, check the patient's standing blood pressure and pulse.

• A standing decrease in systolic blood pressure by 20 mm Hg or more is consistent with orthostatic hypotension; there may or may not be an increase in pulse depending on the cause. Patients whose orthostasis is due to volume depletion would be expected to have the ability to mount a tachycardic response to the blood pressure drop; however, patients with autonomic insufficiency may have profound orthostatic drops in blood pressure with little or no increase in pulse rate. When orthostatic hypotension is found, it is also important to ask the patient if any symptoms during the test re-created his or her presenting complaints.

Imbalance

• In the patient with possible imbalance as the cause of dizziness, pay particular attention to assessing gait and look for abnormalities of motor, sensory, or cerebellar function.
• Look for proprioceptive loss in the toes or a Romberg sign (see Chapter 32, Romberg Testing); however, it is more common to discover subtle Romberg-like findings by history (worsened imbalance in the dark or in the shower) than to detect proprioceptive loss or a Romberg sign on examination. Often, the only examination clue to neuropathic or posterior column dysfunction is vibratory loss in the feet.

Vertigo

• Patients with vertigo due to acute cerebellar or brainstem dysfunction may have significant gait ataxia and may even be unable to walk without assistance (see Chapter 39, Examination of Gait).
• Patients with peripheral vestibular disorders may have some difficulty with gait, particularly while acutely vertiginous, but usually not with the severity of some patients with an acute central (e.g., cerebellar) process. Patients with vestibular problems may feel pulled and lean toward the side of the vestibular dysfunction, but they can still usually walk without a significant problem.
• Nystagmus may be seen with vertigo of central or peripheral origin. Depending on the cause and severity of the problem, nystagmus can be seen in primary gaze (i.e., while the patient is looking forward) or when eye movements are examined (i.e., in horizontal or vertical gaze). Features of nystagmus that are suggestive of central versus peripheral labyrinthine disorders are summarized in Table 44–1. The most important discriminating feature of nystagmus is that purely vertical nystagmus is strongly suggestive of central (cerebellum or brainstem) causes of vertigo.
• Patients whose clinical symptoms suggest BPPV should undergo positional testing with the Dix-Hallpike test (Fig. 44–1). The purpose of the Dix-Hallpike test (also called the *Bárány maneuver* or the *Nylen-Bárány maneuver*) is to look specifically for evidence to support the diagnosis of BPPV in patients who are clinically suspected of having this syndrome based on the history. It is not a general test of vestibular function. To perform the Dix-Hallpike test:
  1. Inform the patient that you'll be attempting to produce the patient's vertigo with the maneuver, ask the patient to try to keep his or her eyes open throughout, and explain the procedure to the patient.
  2. Have the patient sit up on the examining table (or in bed). Make sure the patient is sitting in a position that will allow the head to be extended off of the table when the patient lies down.
  3. Turn the patient's head to the side (right or left) that you think is most likely, by history, to produce vertigo when the patient lies down [i.e., if

TABLE 44-1   Features of Nystagmus of Central versus Peripheral Origin

Localization of Acute Dysfunction	Type of Nystagmus That May Be Present	Direction of Nystagmus[a] in Relation to Direction of Gaze
Central (cerebellum or brainstem)	Vertical or horizontal; may have rotatory component	Nystagmus may change direction with change in direction of gaze (e.g., nystagmus may be left-beating with gaze to the left and right-beating with gaze to the right)[b]
Peripheral (labyrinth)	Usually horizontal; may have rotatory component	Although nystagmus might only be present when looking in one direction, if it is present in both left and right gaze, the nystagmus always beats in the same direction; peripheral nystagmus is most prominent when gazing in the direction of fast phase[c]

[a]The direction of nystagmus is named after the fast phase (the direction it is beating in).
[b]The finding of changing direction of nystagmus with change in gaze is only helpful in supporting a central origin when present; acute cerebellar disorders may cause nystagmus in only one direction of gaze, appearing similar to peripheral nystagmus.
[c]In peripheral vestibular disorders, the direction of the slow phase points to the side of the vestibular lesion.
Adapted from Hotson JR, Baloh RW. Acute vestibular syndrome. *N Engl J Med* 1998;339:680–685.

the patient says that turning his or her head to the right in bed usually provokes vertigo, test the patient initially with the head to the right (Fig. 44–1A)].

4. While holding the patient's head in your hands, rapidly move the patient down to the head-hanging position, all the while keeping his or her head turned to the side (Fig. 44–1B).

5. Observe the patient in that position for at least 10 seconds, watching for a complaint of vertigo. Look at the patient's eyes for nystagmus during this time, especially during any complaint of vertigo. You don't need to check eye movements; just observe the open eyes for the presence of nystagmus.

6. Sit the patient back up.

7. If the initial maneuver brought on vertigo, consider performing the maneuver again, looking for the typical extinction of the response with repeat testing; however, this additional confirmation is usually not necessary.

8. If the initial maneuver did not bring on vertigo, sit the patient back up and repeat the procedure with the head turned in the opposite direction.

• Characteristic abnormalities on the Dix-Hallpike maneuver supportive of a diagnosis of BPPV include the following:

  • Recapitulation of the patient's symptoms of positional vertigo, typically lasting up to approximately 30 seconds. The vertigo experienced by patients with BPPV during the Dix-Hallpike maneuver is usually not subtle; patients with this syndrome are often distressed by the vertigo evoked by this test.

  • A characteristic latency to the onset of the vertigo (and nystagmus) that may be delayed up to 10 seconds.

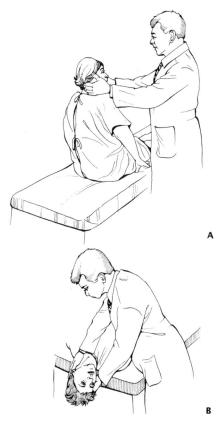

Figure 44-1   Dix-Hallpike testing for benign positional vertigo with the head to the right. See text for details. (Redrawn from Furman JM, Cass SP. Benign paroxysmal positional vertigo. *N Engl J Med* 1999;341:1590–1596.)

- A burst of primarily rotatory (eye rotating toward the dependent ear) nystagmus during the vertigo. The finding of nystagmus, however, although supportive, is of lesser diagnostic importance than the vertigo brought on during the maneuver; this is mainly because it's often hard to visualize the eyes during the patient's distress.
- Extinction of the response [i.e., if the procedure is repeated with the head turned in the same direction, the vertigo (and nystagmus) is less severe].

ADDITIONAL COMMENTS

The distinction between central and peripheral causes of acute vertigo is not always easy on the basis of the history and examination. The finding of brain-stem dysfunction or purely vertical nystagmus strongly supports a central cause, but their absence does not exclude a central (e.g., acute cerebellar) process.

Chapter 45

EXAMINATION OF THE PATIENT WITH HEADACHE

GOAL

The immediate goal of the history and examination of the patient with headache is to determine if the headache potentially represents an urgent or life-threatening process or is a symptom of any other structural brain, meningeal, or systemic process (and, if not, to determine by history which primary headache disorder is likely).

PATHOPHYSIOLOGY OF HEADACHE

Headaches can be broadly classified as *secondary* or *primary*.
- Secondary headaches are due to a structural brain lesion (e.g., tumor), increased intracranial pressure (e.g., tumor or hydrocephalus), a meningeal process (e.g., meningitis or subarachnoid hemorrhage), or systemic illness (e.g., temporal arteritis). These processes produce headache due to irritation of pain-sensitive intracranial (e.g., meninges) or extracranial (e.g., scalp) structures.
- Primary headaches are not due to a structural brain, meningeal, or systemic process. Common primary headaches include migraine, tension, and cluster headache.

TAKING THE HISTORY OF A PATIENT WITH HEADACHE

The history should be obtained with the immediate goal of determining whether the headache is likely to be secondary to a serious process that may require urgent investigation and treatment. The following are some historical clues (summarized in Table 45–1) that are helpful in the clinical assessment of patients with headache:
- Always ask about the onset and time course of development of the headache. Suddenness of headache onset (i.e., an explosive onset developing over seconds) strongly suggests the possibility of aneurysmal subarachnoid (or other intracranial) hemorrhage. Gradually progressive headaches (e.g., over days, weeks, or months) suggest the possibility of intracranial mass lesion, hydrocephalus, or other causes of increased intracranial pressure.
- Ask about symptoms of meningeal irritation (meningismus), such as neck stiffness or photophobia that may be seen in some patients with subarachnoid hemorrhage or meningitis (photophobia is also a common symptom of migraine).
- Ask about any focal neurologic symptoms, such as weakness, double vision, sensory symptoms, or gait problems, that would suggest a focal intracranial lesion. Nausea and vomiting, although nonspecific and common in migraine, can be a symptom of increased intracranial pressure or lesions in the cerebellum.
- In any elderly patient with new-onset headaches, consider the possibility of temporal arteritis. Ask about discomfort or fatigue in the jaw with chewing (jaw claudication), scalp tenderness, transient monocular vision loss,

TABLE 45–1 Symptoms of Some Serious Causes of Headache

Cause of Headache	Time Course of Headache	Typical Associated Symptoms (in Addition to Headache)
Subarachnoid hemorrhage	Sudden onset	Neck pain and stiffness, photophobia
Meningitis	Subacute onset	Fever, neck pain and stiffness, photophobia, sometimes rash (the presence of confusion or aphasia suggests encephalitis) [a]
Intracranial hemorrhage; intraventricular hemorrhage	Sudden onset, may be progressive	Focal neurologic symptoms, nausea and vomiting, gait dysfunction (especially with cerebellar hemorrhage)
Mass lesion	Gradually progressive	Focal neurologic symptoms, nausea and vomiting
Hydrocephalus	Gradually progressive	Nausea and vomiting, possibly gait dysfunction
Pseudotumor cerebri (idiopathic intracranial hypertension)	Gradually progressive, or waxing and waning	Transient visual obscurations, pulsatile tinnitus, obesity
Temporal arteritis	Waxing and waning	Monocular vision loss (transient or persistent), scalp tenderness, jaw claudication, fevers, muscle aches

[a]Meningeal processes can also cause cranial nerve or radicular symptoms due to location of these structures within the subarachnoid space; this most commonly occurs in chronic (e.g., infectious, neoplastic, or inflammatory) meningitides.

constitutional symptoms, or diffuse muscle ache (suggestive of polymyalgia rheumatica).

- Be suspicious for pseudotumor cerebri (idiopathic intracranial hypertension), especially in the context of an overweight woman with persistent headaches. Additional suggestive historical features include brief (seconds) episodes of vision loss that mainly occur with standing (transient visual obscurations) and pulsatile tinnitus, which represents the whooshing of the patient's own heartbeat.
- Historical features suggestive of the most common primary headache syndromes (migraine, tension, and cluster headaches) are summarized in Table 45–2.

EXAMINING THE PATIENT WITH HEADACHE

Patients with primary headache syndromes likely will have normal neurologic examinations. Patients with serious underlying causes of headaches may also have normal neurologic examinations, underscoring the importance of the neurologic history in all patients with headache. The following important clues may be found on examination, however:

- Funduscopic examination (see Chapter 11, Funduscopic Examination) is critical in any patient with headache. The finding of papilledema (see Fig. 11–2) suggests increased intracranial pressure (e.g., due to mass lesions, hydrocephalus, intracranial or subarachnoid hemorrhage, venous sinus thrombosis, or pseudotumor cerebri). In patients with acute headache, another funduscopic finding to look for is retinal (subhyaloid) hemorrhage (see Fig. 11–3), which may be seen in some patients with subarachnoid hemorrhage.

TABLE 45-2 Symptoms of Migraine, Tension, and Cluster Headaches

Headache Type	Headache Location	Time Course	Additional Symptoms That May Be Present
Migraine	Unilateral (e.g., frontotemporal) or bilateral	Hours or days	Nausea and vomiting; photophobia and phonophobia; may prefer to lie in dark, quiet room during attack; may occur with or without visual aura (see Chapter 49, Examination of the Patient with Visual Symptoms) or other transient focal motor, sensory, or language symptoms (see Chapter 48, Examination of the Patient with Transient Focal Neurologic Symptoms)
Tension	Bilateral; typically involves occiput, neck, or around head	Hours or days	Usually none
Cluster	Unilateral, retroorbital; consistently on the same side for each patient	Minutes to hours; may occur multiple times in a day; occurs in clusters with symptom-free periods lasting months to years	Pain is excruciating; may be associated with ipsilateral eye tearing, nasal congestion, rhinorrhea, droopy eyelid during headache; patients often need to get up and pace during an attack

- When subarachnoid hemorrhage or meningitis is a concern, test for nuchal rigidity by gently flexing the patient's neck forward; significant resistance or pain to this maneuver suggests meningitis. Also test for meningismus by checking for Kernig's and Brudzinski's signs, which look for signs of resistance to stretching of nerve roots that have been irritated due to meningeal inflammation.
  - Brudzinski's sign consists of flexion of the hips and legs when you passively flex the patient's neck forward.
  - To test for Kernig's sign, passively flex the patient's hip so that the thigh is held up at approximately 90 degrees, then attempt to passively extend (straighten) the patient's leg at the knee, looking for significant resistance to this maneuver and pain.
- Unilateral pupillary dilation, with or without ipsilateral ptosis or other eye movement findings consistent with a third nerve palsy (see Chapter 10, Examination of the Pupils), suggests a posterior communicating artery aneurysm or other compressive lesion.
- The finding of Horner's syndrome (see Chapter 10, Examination of the Pupils) would suggest carotid dissection or cluster headache (if examined during an attack).
- When temporal arteritis is a consideration, palpate the temporal arteries looking for temporal artery tenderness or induration.
- Any focal findings on the general neurologic examination suggest focal intracranial processes, but their absence does not exclude such processes.

EXAMINATION OF THE PATIENT WITH A MOVEMENT DISORDER

Chapter 46

GOAL

The main goal of the examination of the patient with a movement disorder is to characterize the disorder of increased or decreased movements to better understand the diagnosis and management of the patient's symptoms.

PATHOPHYSIOLOGY OF MOVEMENT DISORDERS

Disorders of movement can be divided into those that cause diminished (hypokinetic) movement and those that cause abnormal (hyperkinetic) involuntary movements.

- The hypokinetic movement disorders comprise mainly Parkinson's disease and other parkinsonian syndromes. Parkinson's disease occurs due to degeneration of substantia nigra neurons in the midbrain that project to the basal ganglia. *Parkinsonism*, on the other hand, is the generic name for any clinical syndrome that includes Parkinson's disease-like symptoms.
- The hyperkinetic movement disorders include tremors, dystonia, chorea, myoclonus, and tic disorders. Some of these symptoms occur due to disorders of basal ganglia (extrapyramidal) function (e.g., chorea, parkinsonian tremors, and, probably, dystonia), and some occur due to disorders of cortical or spinal cord function (e.g., myoclonus), but the pathophysiology of some of the hyperkinetic movement disorders (e.g., essential tremor and tic disorders) remains unclear.

TAKING THE HISTORY OF A PATIENT WITH A MOVEMENT DISORDER

More than any other neurologic disorder, the diagnosis of movement disorders depends primarily on observation of the findings on examination. Nonetheless, like any neurologic disorder, the history is integral to the diagnostic process.

- In any patient with a movement disorder, take a good medication history because many medications can cause extrapyramidal symptoms of parkinsonism, dystonia, and chorea (e.g., neuroleptics and antiemetics), and many can cause or worsen postural tremor (e.g., valproic acid, amiodarone, and lithium). Make sure you ask about past medications and not just medicines the patient is currently taking.
- The family history can give important clues for some of the movement disorders, such as Huntington's disease and familial essential tremor.
- Have the patient describe the abnormal movements, the age of onset (e.g., tic disorders usually begin in childhood), and the course of symptoms (e.g., worsening over time suggests a degenerative disorder).
- Ask about any exacerbating or relieving factors (e.g., essential tremor may be worse with stress and improved with alcohol; patients with cervical dystonia may have found maneuvers to temporarily relieve the symptoms; patients with focal dystonias may only develop their symptoms during certain activities). Ask if there is any control over the movements (e.g., tic disorders).

- Inquire about other associated symptoms that may provide diagnostic clues in the appropriate clinical situations, such as cognitive symptoms (e.g., Huntington's disease and Wilson's disease), autonomic symptoms (e.g., Shy-Drager syndrome), and systemic problems (e.g., liver dysfunction in Wilson's disease or a recent streptococcal infection in Sydenham's chorea).

EXAMINING THE PATIENT WITH A MOVEMENT DISORDER

Parkinsonism

- Parkinson's disease usually presents as asymmetric slowness (bradykinesia), rigidity, and tremors. Other parkinsonian syndromes are more likely to present symmetrically.
- Observe for diminished facial expression consistent with masked facies and listen to the speech, which may be soft and even stuttering in some patients.
- Observe the patient for a resting tremor in the hands, although not all patients have a tremor. The typical parkinsonian tremor is described as *pill-rolling* because of the characteristic oscillating movements between the thumb and the other fingers. It is often asymmetric, especially early in the course of Parkinson's disease, and it tends to occur at rest and diminishes when the arm is performing a task. The tremor may be particularly prominent when the patient is preoccupied with another task, such as walking or manipulating the opposite hand. In some patients, a similar resting tremor may be seen in a foot as it dangles off the examining table.
- Test for cogwheel rigidity as described in Chapter 27, Examination of Tone. The ability to perform fine movements and rapid alternating movements (see Chapter 34, Testing of Upper Extremity Cerebellar Function) may be impaired in parkinsonism due to slowness from basal ganglia dysfunction. Strength should be normal.
- Ask the patient to write a sentence (not their signature); patients with Parkinson's disease usually have small (micrographic), shaky handwriting. Also ask the patient to draw a spiral from the inside out (draw a sample of this for the patient, by drawing a loose spiral a few inches in diameter); patients with Parkinson's disease usually draw a small, tightly packed spiral.
- Examine the gait (see Chapter 39, Examination of Gait) for typical signs of parkinsonism, including diminished arm swing; multiple small, narrow-based, shuffling steps; and a stooped posture. The patient may have difficulty getting up out of a chair to initiate gait. *Festination* of gait refers to the tendency of parkinsonian patients to keep speeding up when walking, with difficulty stopping their forward progress. Make sure you observe the patient turn and walk back to you, because patients with parkinsonism may show typical *en bloc* turning, taking multiple extra steps as they attempt to change direction, rather than a normal pivot. There may also be a tendency to freeze at doorways and with turns.
- In any patient with suspected parkinsonism, assess postural reflexes:
  1. Ask the patient to stand still. Inform the patient that you will be testing balance by pulling him or her backward and that the patient should maintain balance as best as he or she can and may take steps backward if necessary.
  2. Stand directly behind the patient, so if the patient were to fall backward, you would be able catch him or her.

3. Reach around and pull back quickly on the patient's shoulders and observe the patient's ability to retain his or her balance. Obviously, catch the patient if he or she begins to fall into you.
4. Impairment of postural reflexes would manifest as a series of backward steps or as the patient falling backward.

- Patients with the parkinsonian syndrome of progressive supranuclear palsy may have difficulty with voluntary conjugate eye movements (see Chapter 14, Examination of Eye Movements) and especially may have difficulty looking down as the earliest eye sign of the disease. In these patients, the *supranuclear* (i.e., above the cranial nerve nuclei in the brainstem) cause of the dysfunction can usually be detected by finding that the downward eye movements are intact when the patient's head is passively tilted upward while the patient is asked to fixate his or her eyes forward on your face.
- When the Shy-Drager syndrome (a form of multiple-system atrophy) is suspected, be certain to look for evidence of orthostatic hypotension (see Chapter 44, Examination of the Dizzy Patient).

Postural (Essential) Tremor

- Unlike parkinsonian tremors, patients with essential tremor or other postural tremors have a tremor that is worse with activities that involve maintaining their arm in a specific posture or with action, rather than at rest. Holding a cup of coffee or a soup spoon may be difficult and embarrassing to the patient.
- To assess for a postural tremor, have the patient hold his or her hands directly in front with the palms down and fingers spread (abducted), and observe the hands. Depending on the severity, there may be a subtle fine tremor of the fingers or more prominent, higher amplitude shakiness. Giving the patient a cup of water to hold can also be a good way for you to see the real-world severity of the tremor.
- Watch the patient write a sentence of his or her choice. Patients with essential tremor usually have tremulous handwriting that, unlike parkinsonian writing, is not micrographic. Ask the patient to draw a spiral (draw a sample for the patient), which will be shaky but not micrographic as would occur in Parkinson's disease.
- Look for accentuation of essential tremor during the finger-to-nose maneuver (see Chapter 34, Testing of Upper Extremity Cerebellar Function) as an endpoint tremor. This usually manifests as a fine shakiness when the patient's finger gets close to your finger or his or her nose but without the clumsiness (dysmetria) throughout the maneuver seen in cerebellar disorders.

Dystonia

- Dystonic movements are abnormal, sustained muscle contractions that result in abnormal postures. Depending on the syndrome, these dystonic postures may be focal or generalized, and they may involve the limbs, neck, body, or face.
- Patients with dystonia have abnormal postures of the involved body part evident simply by observation during the examination.
- Patients with focal cervical dystonia (torticollis) show abnormal posturing of the neck, resulting in a combination of head turning, tilting, flexion, or extension. The patient may have the ability to prevent the posture by performing a self-learned simple maneuver such as touching the chin (called a *geste antagoniste*).

- Patients with symptoms suggestive of writer's cramp or other focal or occupational dystonias should be observed in the act of performing the inciting activity (such as writing), so that you can observe the dystonic movements.

Chorea

- *Chorea* manifests on examination as rapid, fidgety-appearing movements, primarily of the extremities, but it may also involve the face. These movements, which are often described as dance-like, are not stereotyped and move unpredictably from one area of the body to another (unlike myoclonus or tics).
- Patients with generalized chorea (such as from Huntington's disease) look fidgety and may be misdiagnosed as simply "nervous." Patients with choreiform movements often, probably inadvertently, try to hide their choreiform movements by incorporating them into maneuvers such as brushing their hair with their hand.
- Hemichorea is chorea involving only one side of the body. Hemichorea and *hemiballismus* (defined as flinging movements of the extremities on one side) are essentially clinically indistinguishable from each other.

Tic Disorders

- Tics are rapid, stereotyped movements or vocalizations. Motor tics may involve the face (e.g., eye blinking), head (e.g., shaking), or extremities. Unlike chorea, tics are generally stereotyped for each patient (i.e., the patient usually manifests the same types of behavior intermittently). Vocal tics may be simple sounds (e.g., throat clearing) or more complex vocalizations, including obscenities (coprolalia).
- Patients may be observed to be able to voluntarily suppress the tics at least to some extent, but they usually describe a build-up of tension that is released as they allow the tics to express themselves again.

Myoclonus

The movements of myoclonus are rapid muscle jerks. Myoclonus may be focal, involving a single extremity or part of an extremity, or generalized. Generalized myoclonus is a common clinical finding, especially in patients with metabolic encephalopathies.

ADDITIONAL COMMENTS

- The term *athetosis* is used to describe slow, writhing movements of the extremities. These movements can occur within the context of chorea (hence the common term *choreoathetosis*), but athetosis can also be seen in the setting of dystonia or even peripheral nerve disorders affecting position sense (pseudoathetosis), as described in Chapter 30, Examination of Vibration and Position Sensation.
- Wilson's disease is an important, treatable (but otherwise progressive) cause of a (hypokinetic or hyperkinetic) movement disorder. When this disorder is a consideration, the finding of copper deposition around the edge of the cornea (Kayser-Fleischer rings) needs to be sought on examination, but it requires slit-lamp examination by an ophthalmologist to be observed.

Chapter 47

EXAMINATION OF THE PATIENT WITH A RADICULOPATHY

GOAL

The goal of the history and examination of the patient with a possible radiculopathy is to look for evidence that the patient's symptoms are likely due to nerve root dysfunction and to try to localize the symptoms and signs to the distribution of a particular nerve root.

PATHOPHYSIOLOGY OF RADICULOPATHY

The term *radiculopathy* refers to any cause of nerve root dysfunction, which can occur due to a structural (compressive) process or nonstructural (noncompressive) process.

- Structural causes of radiculopathy include any process that causes mechanical compression of nerve roots, such as herniated discs (most common in the cervical or lumbar spine), degenerative disease of the spine (e.g., spondylosis), or tumor.
- Nonstructural causes of radiculopathy include diabetic radiculopathy, which likely occurs due to infarction of a nerve root (most commonly affecting the thoracic or lumbar nerve roots), or *Herpes zoster*, which causes radiculopathy due to viral-mediated inflammation of a nerve root.

Pathophysiology of Cervical and Lumbar Radiculopathy due to Herniated Discs

- Cervical nerve roots exit the cord to enter their foramen at the disc space above their respective vertebra, where they are vulnerable to compression from disc herniation or foraminal stenosis. For example, the C7 nerve root exits the cord at the C6-C7 disc space level (i.e., above C7) and is susceptible to compression from this disc or by foraminal stenosis at this level.
- Lumbar nerve roots exit the cord to enter their foramen below their respective vertebra. For example, the L5 nerve root exits the cord at the L5-S1 disc space level (i.e., below L5). The root actually exits above the disc, however, so a herniated disc will affect the next root that is descending within the spinal canal to exit at the next foramen. In other words, a herniated disc at the L5-S1 disc level will most likely affect the S1 root, but foraminal stenosis at the L5-S1 intervertebral foramen level will affect the exiting L5 root.

TAKING THE HISTORY OF A PATIENT WITH A RADICULOPATHY

- Radiculopathic pain is characterized by sharp, shooting discomfort, which may include paresthesias or dysesthesias, radiating proximally to distally in the distribution of the affected nerve root. There may or may not be associated neck or back pain.
- Cervical radiculopathies typically begin in the lateral neck/trapezius region, and lumbar radiculopathies typically begin in the buttock/hip region; both radiate downward within the distribution of the affected

TABLE 47-1   Clues to the Localization of Cervical Radiculopathy

Cervical Root Level	Probable Site of Herniated Disc	Distribution of Pain and Paresthesias[a]	Easily Testable Muscles That May Be Affected[b]	Reflex That May Be Diminished[c]
C5	C4-C5	Scapula, deltoid, upper arm	Deltoid, biceps	Biceps
C6	C5-C6[d]	Biceps region, lateral forearm, dorsal thumb and second finger	Biceps, brachioradialis, extensor carpi radialis (wrist extension)	Biceps
C7	C6-C7[d]	Triceps region, dorsal forearm to dorsal third (and possibly also second and fourth) finger(s)	Triceps, extensor digitorum communis (finger extension)	Triceps
C8	C7-T1	Medial (inner) forearm to fifth and fourth fingers	Interossei, finger flexors	Triceps
T1[e]	T1-T2	Axilla to medial (inner) upper arm	Interossei, abductor pollicis brevis (thumb abduction), abductor digiti minimi (little finger abduction)	None

[a]All of the cervical radiculopathies can begin in lateral neck/trapezius/shoulder region before radiating into arm.
[b]See Chapter 25, Examination of Upper Extremity Muscle Strength, for details on testing these muscles.
[c]See Chapter 37, Examination of the Muscle Stretch Reflexes, for details on testing these reflexes.
[d]These are the most common sites for cervical disc herniation.
[e]T1 root lesions are uncommon and are more likely to occur due to lesions other than disc herniation, including other spinal lesions or apical chest lesions (i.e., Pancoast tumor, in which there usually is also ipsilateral Horner's syndrome).

nerve root. Tables 47–1 and 47–2 summarize the clinical features of cervical and lumbar radiculopathies.

- Pain due to cervical and lumbar radiculopathies from herniated discs is often worsened with coughing, sneezing, or other Valsalva maneuvers, so patients should be specifically asked about this.
- Historical clues to the possibility of a noncompressive radiculopathy include a recent rash in the same distribution to suggest *Herpes zoster* or a radiculopathy in an unusual distribution (e.g., a thoracic root) in a patient with diabetes.

EXAMINING THE PATIENT WITH RADICULOPATHY

- Patients with cervical or lumbar radiculopathy may or may not have weakness in the distribution of muscles supplied by the involved nerve root. If weakness is present, the distribution of weakness (Tables 47–1 and 47–2) should aid in the localization of the patient's radiculopathy to a particular root level.

TABLE 47–2   Clues to the Localization of Lumbar Radiculopathy

Lumbar Root Level	Probable Site of Herniated Disc	Distribution of Pain and Paresthesias	Easily Testable Muscles That May Be Affected[a]	Reflex That May Be Diminished[b]
L4[c]	L3-L4	Knee, medial leg, medial ankle, medial foot	Quadriceps (knee extension), tibialis anterior (foot dorsiflexion)	Knee jerk (patellar reflex)
L5	L4-L5[d]	Buttock, posterolateral thigh, anterolateral shin, dorsum of foot, large toe	Tibialis anterior (foot dorsiflexion), extensor hallucis longus (large toe dorsiflexion), peroneus longus (foot eversion), tibialis posterior (foot inversion)[e]	No testable reflex
S1	L5-S1[d]	Buttock, posterior thigh, posterior calf, lateral foot, little toe, sole of foot	Gastrocnemius (plantar flexion)	Ankle jerk (Achilles reflex)

[a]See Chapter 26, Examination of Lower Extremity Muscle Strength, for details on testing these muscles.
[b]See Chapter 37, Examination of the Muscle Stretch Reflexes, for details on testing these reflexes.
[c]This is an uncommon localization for a lumbar radiculopathy.
[d]These are the most common sites for lumbar disc herniation.
[e]The finding of foot inversion weakness is important in clinically differentiating a severe L5 radiculopathy from a peroneal nerve palsy; both can cause foot drop, but inversion of the foot should be spared in a peroneal nerve palsy.

- Although it is common for patients with cervical or lumbar radiculopathy to have paresthesias in the distribution of the affected nerve root, it's less common to find significant sensory loss on examination, probably due to overlap from the dermatomes of adjacent healthy roots. When sensory loss is found, the dermatomal distribution (Fig. 28–1) is helpful as a further clue to localization to a particular root level.
- Patients with cervical or lumbar radiculopathies may have a diminished reflex in the territory of the involved root if a testable reflex is served by that root (see Table 37–2). L5 radiculopathies do not have a testable reflex to aid in localization.
- The diagnosis of lumbar radiculopathies due to herniated discs may be aided by performing the straight-leg-raising test, which causes discomfort due to stretching of the irritated (compressed) lumbar root. To perform this procedure:
  1. Have the patient lie flat on his or her back (supine) on the examining table.
  2. On the side of the probable radiculopathy, slowly lift the patient's leg by holding it up from the ankle, so that you are passively flexing the patient's hip while the leg remains stiff and extended (locked) at the knee.
  3. Note whether there is radiculopathic-type pain or paresthesias as you lift the leg up (a positive straight-leg-raising test), whether it recapitu-

lates the patient's presenting symptoms, and note the approximate angle at which the discomfort occurred. Tightness in the hamstrings when the leg is lifted is normal and not specific for radiculopathy.

• Patients with possible *Herpes zoster* should be examined for a vesicular rash. In any patient with possible radiculopathy from diabetes or *Herpes zoster*, look for cutaneous dysesthesias to gross touch or pinprick in the involved dermatome. This is particularly helpful when a thoracic radiculopathy is present, because pain in this distribution can be confused with a visceral process; the finding of cutaneous dysesthesias or sensory loss is an important clue to a radiculopathic cause of symptoms.

ADDITIONAL COMMENTS

Sciatica is a generic descriptive term referring to any pain radiating within the distribution of the sciatic nerve (i.e., from the buttock down the leg). Patients with symptoms of sciatica are much more likely to have a radiculopathy (affecting the L5 or S1 root) than a lesion of the sciatic nerve.

Chapter 48

EXAMINATION OF THE PATIENT WITH TRANSIENT FOCAL NEUROLOGIC SYMPTOMS

GOAL

The goal of the history and examination of the patient with transient focal neurologic symptoms is to determine the most likely pathophysiology and localization of the patient's symptoms.

PATHOPHYSIOLOGY OF TRANSIENT FOCAL NEUROLOGIC SYMPTOMS

Transient—lasting seconds, minutes, or hours—focal neurologic dysfunction generally occurs as a result of one of three major mechanisms: ischemia, seizure, or migraine.

- Ischemia causes transient focal neurologic symptoms [i.e., transient ischemic attacks (TIAs)] due to diminished blood flow to a focal brain region (see Chapter 52, Examination of the Patient with a Probable Stroke). By definition, a TIA is transient ischemia; a TIA that doesn't resolve is called a *stroke*.
- Partial (also called *focal*) seizure disorders cause transient focal neurologic symptoms due to focal cortical epileptic activity. Partial seizures that do not impair consciousness are called *simple partial seizures*. Partial seizures that impair consciousness (such as many temporal lobe seizures) are called *complex partial seizures*. Partial seizures may spread to involve the whole brain, causing a secondarily generalized seizure (in contrast to a primary generalized seizure, which begins simultaneously on both sides of the brain and does not have a focal onset or focal symptomatology).
- Migraine can cause transient focal neurologic symptoms; the pathogenesis of migrainous neurologic symptoms is uncertain but may be due to a slowly spreading wave of depolarization called *spreading cortical depression*.

TAKING THE HISTORY OF A PATIENT WITH TRANSIENT FOCAL NEUROLOGIC SYMPTOMS

The major clues to the localization and mechanism of the patient's symptoms are likely to be found from a careful neurologic history aimed at listening to the patient's (and witnesses') description of the episodes.

Ischemia

- TIAs usually occur suddenly and last seconds or minutes before resolving.
- Depending on the arterial distribution, ischemia can cause any kind of focal neurologic deficit, such as focal weakness, numbness, vision loss or diplopia, vertigo, aphasia or dysarthria. Listen for the distribution of the patient's symptoms to determine the most likely involved vascular territory (see Chapter 52, Examination of the Patient with a Probable Stroke).
- A history of recurrent, stereotyped TIAs in the same distribution (i.e., the same deficit occurring multiple times over days, weeks, or months) suggests the presence of a focal arterial stenosis rather than a cardioembolic

source (see Chapter 52, Examination of the Patient with a Probable Stroke).

- Ask about any transient monocular visual disturbances consistent with amaurosis fugax that would suggest the possibility of carotid stenosis (see Chapter 49, Examination of the Patient with Visual Symptoms, and Chapter 52, Examination of the Patient with a Probable Stroke).

Seizure

- Take time to ask the patient to report the whole story of their events from beginning to end. Get history from a witness for symptoms the patient may not be aware of, such as lip smacking or automatisms (e.g., picking at the clothes) that may occur while consciousness is impaired during a complex-partial seizure.
- Seizure symptoms are usually stereotypical for each patient. Depending on the location of the focus, seizures may cause motor, somatosensory, visual, olfactory, visceral, or emotional symptoms. Seizures usually cause "positive" symptoms, such as hallucinations or shaking, rather than "negative" symptoms, such as weakness, as expected with ischemia.
- Always ask the patient about the presence of frequent déjà vu phenomena (a sense of familiarity or having done something before), jamais vu (unfamiliarity), or an olfactory aura (hallucination of a smell). These are typical symptoms of temporal lobe seizures, but patients may not volunteer these symptoms unless asked.
- Seizures may begin with one symptom and spread quickly to involve other symptoms and may then generalize to a tonic-clonic seizure. When patients present because of a generalized seizure, inquire about prodromal symptoms suggestive of a focal onset.
- Ask the patient about symptoms that might suggest unrecognized generalized seizures, such as episodes of nocturnal tongue biting or incontinence.

Migraine

- Neurologic symptoms due to migraine may occur with or without headache (see Chapter 45, Examination of the Patient with Headache) or scintillating visual disturbances (see Chapter 49, Examination of the Patient with Visual Symptoms). When present, however, these are helpful clues to a migrainous cause of the patient's symptoms.
- Focal neurologic symptoms from migraine typically march more slowly than symptoms of a seizure; for example, migrainous sensory symptoms may begin with tingling in the hand and slowly spread to the cheek over 15 to 30 minutes. As the symptom progresses, there may even be an associated aphasia or weakness.

EXAMINING THE PATIENT WITH TRANSIENT FOCAL NEUROLOGIC SYMPTOMS

By definition, examination of the patient with transient symptoms is likely to be normal because patients are rarely examined during the deficit. There are a few clues that may be helpful if found, however. For example, when TIA is a consideration, listen for a carotid bruit (see Chapter 52, Examination of the Patient with a Probable Stroke), although this is not a sensitive sign for carotid disease. The presence of any focal findings on examination may suggest a previous infarct in a patient with TIA or may be a clue to an underlying gross structural brain lesion causing seizures.

ADDITIONAL COMMENTS

Multiple sclerosis attacks generally do not cause transient symptoms in the sense described earlier; neurologic dysfunction from exacerbations of multiple sclerosis tends to last days, weeks, or even months before resolving. Transient symptoms can occur in multiple sclerosis due to short circuits through demyelinated lesions, however. These symptoms are often painful, repetitive, brief (seconds), and stereotypical for an individual patient, and they may manifest as tingling, flexion (flexor spasms), or extension (painful tonic spasms) of a limb.

Chapter 49

EXAMINATION OF THE PATIENT WITH VISUAL SYMPTOMS

GOAL

The goal of the history and examination of the patient with visual symptoms is to determine whether the symptoms are due to vision loss or diplopia and to determine the most likely cause of that dysfunction.

PATHOPHYSIOLOGY OF VISUAL DYSFUNCTION

Visual dysfunction, whether transient or persistent, can occur as a result of one of two main mechanisms: *vision loss* or *diplopia.*

- Vision loss can occur due to dysfunction anywhere along the sensory visual pathway that begins in the eyes and ends in the occipital cortex (see Chapter 13, Visual Field Examination, and Fig. 13–1).
- Diplopia is the illusion of seeing two objects when there is really only one and occurs when there is dysfunction of normal conjugate eye movements so that the eyes no longer move appropriately in synchrony. The presence of diplopia implies dysfunction of the motor pathways that move the eyes, anywhere from the brainstem to the extraocular muscles. Because the illusion of diplopia requires two eyes, patients who are blind in one eye cannot have diplopia.

TAKING THE HISTORY OF A PATIENT WITH VISUAL DYSFUNCTION

Listed below are important features of the history that can be helpful in the evaluation of patients who present with symptoms due to vision loss or diplopia.

Vision Loss

Monocular Vision Loss

- *Monocular vision loss* may be transient or persistent. When patients present with transient visual symptoms that they attribute to one eye, for you to be more certain that your patient's symptom was truly monocular and not a hemianopic disturbance, the patient would have had to have covered the bad eye during the event to confirm that the vision was intact in the good eye. Some patients do initiate this test on their own during an episode of vision loss, but you may need to specifically inquire if the patient did this.
- Patients with monocular visual problems do not usually present with significant functional deficits from their vision loss, as long as the remaining eye has intact visual fields. In other words, unlike patients with hemianopsias, patients with purely monocular vision loss are less likely to bump into objects because of their visual dysfunction.
- Amaurosis fugax (meaning *fleeting blindness*) is an important kind of transient monocular vision loss that may be seen in patients with retinal ischemia, such as can be associated with carotid stenosis or temporal arteritis. Patients describe a brief (seconds or minutes) loss of vision in

one eye as "like a shade coming down." As the symptoms resolve, the patient may describe the shade coming back up.

- Patients with optic neuritis usually present with monocular vision loss that progresses over a period of days and lasts for weeks, and it is often associated with pain on eye movement.

Visual Field Loss

- Patients with *visual field loss* often do not recognize the concept of a visual field or a visual field deficit. They may misinterpret their homonymous visual field deficits as monocular (i.e., a patient may interpret a left homonymous hemianopsia as a visual problem involving the left eye alone).
- Patients with hemianopic visual field cuts sometimes present with symptoms of the consequences of their deficits, rather than with a primary visual complaint. They may tell you they consistently bump into objects on one side, or they may have been involved in a motor vehicle collision because of their visual deficit.
- Patients with hemianopsias may present with a vague visual complaint that they have difficulty describing. Those with left homonymous hemianopsias may complain of difficulty reading, not recognizing that their difficulty is due to consistently missing the first (left) parts of sentences. Patients with bitemporal field loss may complain of difficulty with their peripheral vision.
- A common form of transient hemianopic field deficit is the visual disturbance of a migraine aura. Migrainous visual disturbances typically present as a scintillating (shining) zigzag or herringbone-like pattern, sometimes in the form of a C, occurring in the left or right visual field and gradually growing over approximately a 15-minute period before resolving. This migrainous visual disturbance may or may not be followed by a headache.
- Patients with complete bilateral vision loss due to bilateral occipital lobe infarcts can actually be unaware that they are blind and deny the existence of their blindness. This is known as *Anton's syndrome.*

Diplopia

- Patients with diplopia usually are aware of seeing two objects, which (depending on the cause) can be side by side, vertical, or diagonal. Horizontal diplopia would be particularly likely from sixth nerve lesions or disorders affecting the lateral or medial rectus muscles alone. Vertical or diagonal diplopia would be expected with lesions causing the eyes to diverge vertically or diagonally but is otherwise not specific in terms of localization.
- Diplopia should completely resolve when the patient covers either eye. Some patients instinctively perform this test themselves, but you may need to specifically ask if they did, especially if the diplopia was transient and is no longer present during your examination.
- Some patients who have diplopia complain only of a vague blurriness of vision, unaware that their difficulty is actually due to two partially superimposed images. In this case, the historical clue that the visual symptom is actually diplopia rests on the finding that the symptoms resolve with covering either eye.
- Diplopia due to myasthenia gravis usually waxes and wanes like any other weakness associated with this neuromuscular junction disease. The diplopia may be worse at the end of the day and may be associated with eyelid drooping.

EXAMINING THE PATIENT WITH VISUAL DYSFUNCTION

The following are important features of the examination of patients who present with symptoms due to vision loss or diplopia:

Vision Loss

Monocular Vision Loss

- In patients with monocular vision loss due to optic nerve dysfunction (such as optic neuritis), the visual field in the affected eye may be a central scotoma. This is easily detected by asking the patient to cover the good eye and look directly at your face with the bad eye. The patient with a central scotoma describes inability to see the central part of your face but is able to see the periphery.
- On pupillary examination, patients with monocular vision loss due to optic nerve dysfunction also usually have an afferent pupillary defect (see Chapter 10, Examination of the Pupils).
- Acute monocular vision loss due to optic nerve demyelination or inflammation may be associated with optic disc swelling (see Fig. 11–2) if the process involves the optic nerve head itself (papillitis); however, the optic disc will appear normal if the disease process is behind the eye (retrobulbar optic neuritis). Long-standing monocular vision loss from severe optic nerve dysfunction is often associated with significant pallor of the optic disc due to optic nerve atrophy (see Fig. 11–4).
- Patients with transient monocular vision loss (amaurosis fugax) from carotid stenosis may or may not have other evidence for carotid disease on examination, such as a bruit. They may also rarely have refractile (bright) embolic material at the branch points of one or several retinal arterioles visible on funduscopy, called *Hollenhorst plaques* (Fig. 49–1).

Hemianopsia

- In patients with symptoms suggestive of a visual field cut, confrontational visual field testing (see Chapter 13, Visual Field Examination) will usually easily detect a deficit (i.e., a left or right homonymous hemianopsia, quadrantanopsia, or bitemporal hemianopsia).
- Pupillary responses should be normal in patients with hemianopic visual field deficits (as well as in patients with complete vision loss due to bilateral occipital pathology) because the lesion is posterior to the optic chiasm.

Diplopia

- While examining a patient with diplopia, ask the patient to describe the characteristics of the two images to you. This may require the patient to look at an object in the room and tell you whether the two images are side by side (horizontal diplopia), up and down (vertical diplopia), or diagonal.
- Confirm that the diplopia resolves when the patient covers either eye; this simply further confirms that the patient's symptoms fit with diplopia.
- Look at the resting position of the eyes as the patient looks straight ahead. The affected eye of patients with third nerve palsies, for example, characteristically deviates laterally and downward (see Fig. 10–1).

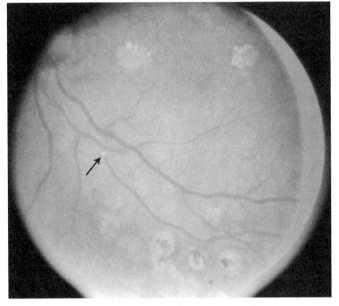

Figure 49–1 Retinal artery embolus (*arrow*) in a patient with carotid atherosclerosis.

- Look closely at the extraocular movements. Particularly, look for evidence of a third or sixth cranial nerve palsy (see Chapter 14, Examination of Eye Movements), and look for pupillary findings suggestive of a third nerve palsy (see Chapter 10, Examination of the Pupils). Also look for evidence of an internuclear ophthalmoplegia (see Fig. 14–2).

- Patients with fourth nerve palsies are recognized more by the characteristic head tilt they adopt (as a compensation for the diplopia that would occur if they didn't hold their head in that position) than the subtle eye movement changes that would be expected from weakness of the superior oblique muscle. Patients with fourth nerve palsies usually tilt their head away from the side of the fourth nerve lesion (i.e., a left fourth nerve palsy would likely cause a head tilt to the right).

- The finding of proptosis in a patient with diplopia suggests that the lesion is within the orbit or involves the eye muscle itself.

- If myasthenia gravis is suspected as a cause of diplopia, look for fatigability of the eye muscles as follows:
  1. Ask the patient to follow your finger with his or her eyes upward as you raise your finger up to test upward gaze.
  2. Continue holding your finger above the patient's head as you observe the patient perform a prolonged upgaze. Watch for a minute or two (your arm may get tired before the patient does) while you observe the patient's eyes.
  3. Weakness of the patient's sustained upgaze would manifest as drifting of one or both of the eyes downward (not just difficulty persisting with

upgaze due to getting tired of the procedure). Also observe for any ptosis of either eye (or worsening ptosis if ptosis is already present).
4. The finding of fatigability of upgaze or worsening ptosis with this procedure can be a helpful clue to the diagnosis of myasthenia gravis even
if eye muscle weakness or ptosis is not seen on routine testing.

Chapter 50

EXAMINATION OF THE PATIENT WITH WEAKNESS OR SENSORY LOSS

GOAL

The goal of examining the patient with weakness or sensory loss is to try to determine the localization and mechanism of the neurologic problem causing the symptoms.

PATHOPHYSIOLOGY

Weakness

The basic neuroanatomy of the motor pathways in the central and peripheral nervous system is outlined in Chapter 24, Approach to the Motor Examination. Weakness can occur due to any kind of lesion affecting the upper motor neuron within the brain or spinal cord, or affecting the lower motor anywhere from the anterior horn cells of spinal cord to the nerve roots, plexus, peripheral nerves, neuromuscular junction, or muscles. Note that the term *weakness* here means any true muscle weakness less than 5 out of 5 (see Chapter 24, Approach to the Motor Examination) and not a subjective generalized sense of fatigue (also called *asthenia*); fatigue is a nonspecific and nonlocalizing symptom that can be seen in many systemic and neurologic illnesses.

Sensory Loss

The basic neuroanatomy of the sensory pathways in the central and peripheral nervous system is outlined in Chapter 28, Approach to the Sensory Examination. Sensory symptoms (such as numbness and tingling) can occur due to any kind of lesion affecting the sensory pathways in the central or peripheral nervous system.

TAKING THE HISTORY OF A PATIENT WITH WEAKNESS OR SENSORY LOSS

The history of the patient with a complaint of weakness or sensory loss should be obtained with the goal of looking for additional clues that may help you determine the localization and mechanism of the problem.

- For a complaint of weakness, during the history, try to pinpoint the areas involved in the weakness (e.g., which extremities are weak or which movements of an extremity are weak), because lesions in various regions of the central and peripheral nervous system produce characteristic patterns of weakness (see Table 24–3). For example, weakness of one side of the body suggests the possibility of a contralateral cerebral hemispheric localization, whereas distal weakness in the lower extremities suggests the possibility of a peripheral neuropathic process. When neuromuscular junction disease (i.e., myasthenia gravis) is a consideration, make sure to ask about any waxing and waning of the weakness, especially worsening at the end of the day, as well as any symptoms of dysarthria, dysphagia, ptosis, or diplopia.

- For a complaint of sensory loss, ask the patient to point to the area or areas involved, because lesions in various regions of the central and peripheral nervous system produce characteristic patterns of sensory loss (see Table 28–2). For example, analogous to weakness, numbness of one side of the body suggests the possibility of a contralateral cerebral hemispheric (or thalamic) localization, whereas distal numbness in the lower extremities suggests the possibility of a peripheral neuropathic process.
- Ask questions during the history with the intent of determining whether there are any additional nonmotor or nonsensory symptoms (such as speech problems, headache, dizziness, visual changes, and bowel or bladder dysfunction) that would further localize the problem to a particular area of the central or the peripheral nervous system (see Table 2–2).
- As in any neurologic history, ask about the temporal pattern of symptom development, which may help you determine the most likely mechanisms of the dysfunction (see Table 3–2).

EXAMINING THE PATIENT WITH WEAKNESS OR SENSORY LOSS

- While examining any patient with a complaint of weakness or sensory loss, make sure that the patient's arms and legs are visible (i.e., he or she should be wearing a hospital gown). For the patient with weakness, this allows you to see atrophy or fasciculations that would be consistent with a lower motor neuron process. For the patient with sensory loss, this allows you to do a more careful sensory examination, not necessarily restricted to the distal extremities.
- In any patient with weakness, do a thorough screen of motor strength testing of proximal and distal muscles of the upper and lower extremities (see the suggested general list of muscles to test in Chapter 40, Performing a Complete Neurologic Examination). Obviously, don't forget to test the extremities and muscles in which the patient specifically complains of weakness.
- In any patient with sensory symptoms, test sensation to pinprick (see Chapter 29, Examination of Pinprick Sensation), as well as to vibration and proprioception (see Chapter 30, Examination of Vibration and Position Sensation); occasionally, cortical sensation (see Chapter 31, Examination of Cortical Sensation) may be helpful in situations in which a right hemispheric localization is suggested.
- Depending on your suspicion as it evolves from the history and during the examination, hone your examination to try to look for characteristic distributions of weakness (see Table 24–3) or sensation (see Table 28–2) to pinpoint the most likely localization of your patient's problem. For example, in the motor examination of a patient in whom you suspect a radial nerve lesion, look for weakness in other radial nerve–innervated muscles and look for preserved strength in nonradial nerve–innervated muscles, even those that share similar nerve root innervation as the weak muscles. In the sensory examination of a patient in whom you suspect a radial nerve lesion, look for sensory loss in the distribution of this nerve with normal sensation elsewhere.
- Be aware that many lesions would be expected, by virtue of their localization, to cause both motor and sensory findings on examination. Such lesions often do not cause proportional changes in motor and sensory function, however, and even lesions that would be expected to cause dysfunction of both may cause predominant or only motor or sensory find-

ings. For example, peripheral polyneuropathies most frequently cause only distal sensory symptoms, and only when severe is distal motor weakness evident.

- Look for significantly hyperactive or hypoactive deep tendon reflexes, hypertonia (or hypotonia), or a Babinski sign (see Table 36–1) to support an upper motor neuron or lower motor neuron localization of your patient's symptoms, and look for characteristic distributions of those reflex findings that would suggest particular localizations (see Tables 36–1 and 37–2).

- In addition to the motor, sensory, and reflex changes described above, throughout your complete neurologic examination, look for any additional findings that would further localize the problem to a particular area of the central or the peripheral nervous system (see Table 2–2).

- The assessment of weakness or sensory loss due to spinal cord dysfunction is discussed in more detail in Chapter 51, Examination of the Patient with a Suspected Spinal Cord Problem, and that due to radiculopathy is discussed in more detail in Chapter 47, Examination of the Patient with a Radiculopathy.

- The clinical diagnosis of a focal peripheral nerve entrapment neuropathy can be aided by looking for Tinel's sign. Tinel's sign is a sensation of tingling in the distribution of a nerve when the involved region of nerve is lightly tapped with your finger or reflex hammer (the funny bone sensation that we've all felt from an impact on our ulnar nerves at the elbows is Tinel's sign). In suspected carpal tunnel syndrome, test for Tinel's sign by tapping over the distal volar wrist in the midline, looking for tingling into the median nerve–innervated fingers. Although not a very sensitive sign, the finding of Tinel's sign in the region of any clinically suspected entrapment neuropathy can be a useful supportive clue to the diagnosis.

- See Chapter 24, Approach to the Motor Examination, and Chapter 28, Approach to the Sensory Examiniation, for further details regarding the evaluation of patients with weakness or sensory loss.

Chapter 51

EXAMINATION OF THE PATIENT WITH A SUSPECTED SPINAL CORD PROBLEM

GOAL

The goal is to recognize, on the basis of the history and examination, when a patient's symptoms are likely to be due to spinal cord dysfunction so that the appropriate investigations can be performed.

PATHOPHYSIOLOGY OF SPINAL CORD DYSFUNCTION

Spinal cord dysfunction can occur due to a compressive lesion extrinsic to the spinal cord (e.g., tumor, abscess, or disc) or due to an intrinsic lesion within the spinal cord (e.g., demyelination, inflammation, or infarction). Dysfunction of the spinal cord due to any cause is referred to by the generic term *myelopathy*. Acute dysfunction of the spinal cord causing severe motor and sensory loss below the level of the lesion is often called a *transverse myelopathy*. When spinal cord dysfunction is thought to be due to an intrinsic demyelinative or inflammatory process, it is called *myelitis*.

Spinal cord dysfunction generally causes motor, sensory, or autonomic dysfunction below the level of the spinal cord lesion; however, the symptoms of spinal cord disease vary, not only depending on the level of the lesion (e.g., cervical or thoracic), but also the severity of the process and the part of the cord that is being affected at that level (Table 51–1).

TAKING THE HISTORY OF A PATIENT WITH A SUSPECTED SPINAL CORD PROBLEM

- When taking the history, use the combination of motor, sensory, and any autonomic (bowel, bladder, sexual) symptoms to clue you in on the possibility that your patient's symptoms might be due to spinal cord dysfunction. Be aware that cord lesions can present in several different ways (Table 51–1).
- Ask about bowel, bladder, and sexual function (patients may not always volunteer this information); these can be affected by lesions at any level of the spinal cord.
- Patients with a lesion at the level of the cervical spinal cord will most likely have symptoms of weakness and sensory loss in the arms and legs; however, mild or moderate cervical spinal cord dysfunction might cause primarily lower extremity symptoms. Patients with lesions at the level of the thoracic cord can have weakness and sensory loss in the legs, trunk, or abdomen below the dermatomal level of the lesion, but they would not have symptoms in the arms.
- Patients who have hemi-spinal cord dysfunction (i.e., dysfunction affecting only the left or right side of the spinal cord at a particular level) may specifically complain of weakness on one side of the body with sensory loss to temperature sensation (such as when taking a shower or bath) on

TABLE 51-1 Signs and Symptoms of Common Spinal Cord Syndromes and the Cauda Equina Syndrome

Spinal Cord Syndrome	Comments	Signs and Symptoms
Transverse myelopathy	Acute severe bilateral spinal cord dysfunction at a level; may occur due to compression, ischemia, or inflammation/demyelination (transverse myelitis)	Severe weakness, sensory loss, bowel and bladder dysfunction, and upper motor neuron signs below level of lesion.
Brown-Séquard syndrome	Hemi-spinal cord dysfunction; can occur due to intrinsic or extrinsic lesions affecting one side of cord more than the other	Weakness, diminished vibration and proprioception, and upper motor neuron signs on the same side of the lesion below the level of lesion; diminished pin and temperature sensation on the side opposite the lesion below the level of the lesion.
Anterior spinal artery syndrome	Due to infarct in distribution of anterior spinal artery; affects the corticospinal and spinothalamic tracts, sparing the posterior columns	Weakness and diminished pinprick sensation (and upper motor neuron signs) below the level of the lesion; vibration and position sense spared.
Cervical syrinx	Due to cavitary lesion within the center of the cervical cord primarily initially affecting the crossing fibers of spinothalamic tract; may also affect anterior horn cells, causing lower motor neuron dysfunction in hands	Diminished pin and temperature sensation in the hands and arms, possibly also the shoulders and chest (cape distribution); may have atrophy and weakness in hands.
Central (cervical) cord syndrome	Dysfunction primarily involving center of cervical cord (acting physiologically like a large syrinx); may occur due to intrinsic cord lesions or compressive lesions	Weakness in the arms more than legs; upper motor neuron signs and posterior column loss primarily in legs; pin sensation loss may be seen in arms and legs, but sacral sensation may be spared.
Conus medullaris syndrome	Dysfunction of the tip of the spinal cord, affecting sacral motor (autonomic) and sensory fibers	Perianal (sacral) sensory loss; incontinence of bowel and bladder; loss of anal sphincter tone.
Cauda equina syndrome	Dysfunction of nerve roots in the lumbosacral spinal canal below L-2 usually due to compressive lesions of the lumbosacral spine	Weakness and sensory loss in legs below the level of the lesion; loss of bowel and bladder function (flaccid and areflexic). Because only lower motor neurons (nerve roots) are affected, no upper motor neuron signs should be seen.

the opposite side of the body, symptoms characteristic of the Brown-Séquard syndrome (Table 51–1).

- Some patients with a myelopathy have Lhermitte's sign, an uncomfortable feeling of electricity, vibration, or tingling radiating down the neck, back, or extremities occurring on neck flexion. Lhermitte's sign is actually a symptom, and not a sign tested for during the examination. Although often primarily thought of as a symptom of spinal cord dysfunction due to multiple sclerosis, Lhermitte's sign can occur due to any process affecting the cervical cord (whether intrinsic or compressive), causing dysfunction of the posterior columns. Lhermitte's sign can be a helpful clue to a cervical spinal cord localization of pathology; therefore, patients with a suspicion of spinal cord dysfunction should specifically be asked about the presence or absence of this symptom.

- Most patients with spinal cord dysfunction do not have pain in the neck or back. Neck or back pain may occur in some patients with spinal cord disorders, however, particularly those with epidural spinal cord compression from neoplasms or abscesses that are also affecting bone. Radicular pain may occur in patients who have pathology causing simultaneous root and cord dysfunction.

- Like any neurologic process, the temporal course of symptom development can provide clues to the most likely mechanism of the cord dysfunction. Sudden dysfunction suggests acute compression or infarction, whereas more gradually progressive symptoms suggest processes such as chronic compression, inflammation, or demyelination.

EXAMINING THE PATIENT WITH SUSPECTED SPINAL CORD DYSFUNCTION

- The motor examination of patients with spinal cord disorders may show weakness in muscles below the level of the cord lesion. Depending on the severity of the process, the weakness may be mild or severe. The highest level of major root innervation of the weak muscles (see Tables 25–1 and 26–1) represents the lowest possible superior aspect of the spinal cord lesion. In other words, if there is weakness in C6–innervated muscles and below, the spinal cord lesion must start at or above C6.

- The sensory examination of a patient with spinal cord dysfunction may show bilateral sensory loss to any modality below the level of the lesion. Sensory testing should particularly focus on looking for diminished pin sensation below a dermatomal level, by marching the pin down from superior to inferior dermatomes on each side of the body, asking the patient if there is any decrease in the pin sensation as you go down. March the pin down the chest and abdomen when assessing for a thoracic pin sensation level or between dermatomes of the arm looking for a cervical pin level. If a sensory level is found, the pin level represents the lowest possible superior aspect of the spinal cord lesion. In other words, if there is diminished pin sensation from the T4 level and down (i.e., normal above T4), the spinal cord lesion must start at or somewhere above T4. Cervical cord lesions may, therefore, sometimes cause a thoracic sensory level.

- The sensory examination of patients with spinal cord disorders usually also shows loss of vibration sensation (and, if severe, proprioceptive loss) below the level of the lesion. These signs of posterior column dysfunction are helpful in assessing the severity of a lesion (i.e., the more severe the lesion, the worse the vibration or proprioceptive sensation loss below the lesion) but are not as helpful in defining the possible level of the lesion as pin sensation.

- Patients with spinal cord dysfunction typically have upper motor neuron signs (hyperreflexia) below the level of the lesion, as well as upgoing toes (Babinski sign). Patients with chronic spinal cord disorders also typically have increased tone (spasticity) below the level of the lesion.

- When a hemi-spinal cord (Brown-Séquard) syndrome is suspected, in addition to assessing for asymmetric weakness, look for side-to-side differences in vibration and proprioception, as well as side-to-side differences in pin and temperature sensation below the level of the lesion. To test temperature sensation, simply touch an area of skin on each side of the patient's body with the side of a (nonvibrating) tuning fork, because a metal tuning fork usually feels cold against the skin. Ask the patient if he or she feels the coldness the same on each side. A sensory level to temperature sensation can also be tested in the Brown-Séquard syndrome (or in any potential spinal cord syndrome) simply by marching the side of the tuning fork from superior dermatomes down to inferior dermatomes.
- Anal sphincter tone should be examined in patients when a significant spinal cord disorder (particularly due to possible spinal cord compression) is suspected. Sphincter tone can be assessed by performing a digital lubricated rectal examination and feeling the resistance to insertion of your finger during insertion and after asking the patient to squeeze down. Any decrease you perceive in sphincter tone is potentially abnormal. Another test of sphincter function that may be helpful in the assessment of severe spinal cord disorders is the anal wink reflex. This consists of stroking the perianal skin lightly with a wooden stick and looking for reflex contraction of the anal sphincter; this reflex can be lost with severe spinal cord disorders.
- Table 51–1 summarizes the characteristic signs and symptoms of various common spinal cord syndromes, as well as the cauda equina syndrome (due to lesions affecting the lumbosacral roots below the spinal cord).

Chapter 52

EXAMINATION OF THE PATIENT WITH A PROBABLE STROKE

GOAL

The main goal of the examination of the patient with a probable stroke is to try to determine the most likely location in the brain (and, therefore, the most likely vascular distribution) where the stroke occurred, as well as the most likely pathogenesis of the stroke, paving the way for the most appropriate investigation and management.

PATHOPHYSIOLOGY OF STROKE

A *stroke* is acute destruction of brain tissue occurring from infarction or hemorrhage.

Cerebral Infarction

- Infarction can occur due to stenosis or occlusion of a blood vessel from disease or thrombosis within the vessel itself (referred to here as *intrinsic cerebrovascular disease*) or embolism from a proximal source, such as the heart (*cardioembolism*). Embolism from an artery to an artery can also occur (such as distal embolism from a carotid plaque), but it is helpful to think of artery-to-artery embolism within the spectrum of intrinsic cerebrovascular disease.
- Intrinsic cerebrovascular disease can involve large (e.g., carotid, vertebral, or basilar) arteries, medium (e.g., middle and anterior cerebral) arteries, or small (e.g., lenticulostriate or other small end vessels) arteries of the anterior or posterior circulation.
- Strokes due to intrinsic disease of large or medium-sized blood vessels or strokes due to cardioembolism may involve the cerebral cortex or deeper structures. Strokes due to disease of small blood vessels, such as lacunar strokes (seen in patients with small vessel disease from hypertension or diabetes), only involve deep brain structures and don't involve the cortex. In other words, hemispheric infarcts that involve the cortex can't be due to small vessel disease.

Cerebral Hemorrhage

Hemorrhage within the substance of the brain, called *intraparenchymal* or *intracerebral hemorrhage*, occurs due to rupture of a vessel within the brain. Intraparenchymal hemorrhages and ischemic infarcts are usually indistinguishable on clinical grounds alone, and any patient who presents with an acute stroke syndrome could potentially have a hemorrhagic or ischemic etiology of the event. Intracerebral hemorrhages are usually easily acutely visualized on imaging, such as computed tomography scanning, however. Because the presence and cause of acute ischemic strokes are not always immediately obvious, this chapter focuses on the clinical role of the history and examination in ischemic stroke diagnosis.

TAKING THE HISTORY OF A PATIENT WITH A STROKE

The history and examination are performed to attempt to determine the general vascular distribution in which the stroke occurred and the most likely pathophysiology of the stroke.

Using the History to Determine Stroke Localization

Use the history to try to generate a hypothesis as to the most likely gross anatomic localization of the stroke based on the symptoms of the deficit. Don't be too fancy or try to overlocalize. Be happy if, after the history is obtained, you have a pretty good idea as to whether the stroke is in the left hemisphere (deep or cortical), right hemisphere (deep or cortical), brainstem, or cerebellum. The following are historical features helpful in stroke localization:

- Don't forget to ask if your patient is right- or left-handed, because symptoms of aphasia from left hemispheric cortical lesions or neglect from right hemispheric lesions are less likely to occur in left-handed patients.
- Symptoms of weakness or numbness of the right side of the body (especially of the face and arm, with or without leg weakness) suggest a lesion of the left hemisphere, which could be deep or cortical. A cortical localization of a left hemisphere stroke is suggested by the presence of aphasia, which may be evident while the history is being taken.
- Symptoms of weakness or numbness of the left side of the body (especially of the face and arm, with or without leg weakness) suggest a lesion of the right hemisphere, which could be deep or cortical. A cortical localization of a right hemisphere stroke is suggested during the history by the patient's denial of the left-sided deficit (anosognosia) or left-sided neglect, such as the patient's failure to dress the left side of the body (dressing apraxia).
- Symptoms of a brainstem stroke can include double vision, nausea, vomiting, weakness (which can be unilateral or bilateral), numbness (which also can be unilateral or bilateral), clumsiness, unsteadiness, and vertigo. Crossed symptoms, such as weakness or numbness on one side of the face and the opposite side of the body, can also be seen due to some brainstem infarcts.
- Symptoms of a cerebellar stroke include clumsiness, unsteadiness, vertigo, nausea, vomiting, and, sometimes, headache. Weakness and sensory loss are not accompaniments of an isolated cerebellar stroke.
- Symptoms of visual field loss (hemianopsia) can occur with strokes in the anterior or the posterior circulation. Prominent isolated visual field symptoms, however, are more likely to occur due to strokes involving the posterior circulation involving the occipital cortex (posterior cerebral artery territory).

Using the History to Determine the Stroke Mechanism

The temporal course of symptom development, as well as the presence of any previous symptoms, such as transient ischemic attacks (TIAs), can provide useful information as to the most likely cause of an ischemic stroke (Table 52–1).

- Intrinsic vascular disease is the most likely cause of ischemic stroke when symptoms are gradual or when there are preceding symptoms consistent with TIAs in the same vascular distribution. Patients who present with a history of multiple TIAs in the same distribution of the stroke are espe-

TABLE 52-1 Historical Clues to Ischemic Stroke Mechanism Based on Temporal Course of Symptoms or the Presence of Preceding Symptoms

Symptoms	Most Likely Stroke Mechanism	Least Likely Stroke Mechanism
Gradual progression	Intrinsic vascular disease	Cardioembolism
Sudden onset	Cardioembolism or intrinsic vascular disease	Stroke of any mechanism can be sudden in onset
Recent transient ischemic attacks in same vascular territory as the stroke	Intrinsic vascular disease	Cardioembolism
Recent amaurosis fugax in eye on same side as current brain dysfunction	Intrinsic vascular disease involving carotid artery	Cardioembolism, medium or small vessel disease
Previous transient ischemic attacks in multiple vascular territories	Cardioembolism	Intrinsic vascular disease

cially unlikely to have a cardiogenic embolic cause, given the low probability of multiple emboli from the heart repeatedly entering a single vascular distribution.

- Cardiogenic embolic strokes typically cause sudden symptoms; however, sudden symptoms can also occur due to strokes from intrinsic vascular disease (or from hemorrhage).
- Symptoms of cortical dysfunction in a patient with a hemispheric infarct suggest that the stroke is due to intrinsic large or medium-sized vessel disease or due to cardiogenic embolism, and not due to small vessel disease. The absence of cortical involvement, however, doesn't exclude a large vessel or cardiac cause.
- Ask the patient specifically about any symptoms of monocular vision loss consistent with amaurosis fugax (see Chapter 49, Examination of the Patient with Visual Symptoms). Patients with such visual symptoms often don't recognize their significance, and they are unlikely to volunteer the information because they often assume it is irrelevant to their presenting stroke symptoms. A history consistent with amaurosis fugax of the eye on the same side as the current brain dysfunction (i.e., opposite to the weak extremities) is highly suggestive of the possibility of an extracranial carotid stenosis.
- Use the patient's past medical history to assess for risk factors for intrinsic vascular disease or thrombosis (e.g., diabetes, hypertension, coronary artery disease, peripheral vascular disease, hypercoagulable states) or risk factors for cardioembolism (e.g., atrial fibrillation, cardiomyopathy, valvular disease). The presence of a risk factor for a particular stroke etiology should not supersede the other elements of the patient's history in determining the likely stroke mechanism, however. For example, even in a patient with atrial fibrillation, a stroke that was preceded by multiple TIAs in the same distribution of the stroke is more likely to be due to intrinsic vascular disease than cardioembolism.
- In the emergency evaluation of a patient with a probable acute ischemic stroke, it's also important to determine the time of onset of the stroke, although this does not provide information regarding the pathophysio-

logic stroke mechanism. The timing is especially important when intervention with intravenous tissue plasminogen activator is a consideration, because this medication needs to be given within 3 hours of ischemic stroke onset. The time of stroke symptom onset is defined as the last time the patient was known to be without the stroke symptoms. If a patient awakens with a stroke, the time of onset must be considered the time the patient went to sleep.

EXAMINING THE PATIENT WITH A STROKE

After completing the history, use the examination to help confirm, refute, or refine your hypothesis regarding your patient's stroke localization and mechanism. In addition to the routine general and neurologic examinations (see Chapter 40, Performing a Complete Neurologic Examination), the specific elements listed below may be of particular value in the evaluation of patients with possible stroke.

Carotid Examination

- Listen for carotid bruits. Although the finding of a carotid bruit is useful evidence for the presence of carotid artery disease, the absence of a bruit does not exclude it. To listen for a bruit:
  1. Place your stethoscope on one side of the patient's neck.
  2. Ask the patient to hold his or her breath or to breathe quietly while you listen.
  3. If you hear a bruit, try to confirm that the sound you're hearing doesn't represent a transmitted cardiac murmur. To do this, listen to the heart, the aortic area, and then the neck again. A sound heard primarily over the carotid area but not over the other regions is most suggestive that the bruit is of carotid origin.
  4. Repeat the same on the other side of the neck.
- In neurologic diagnosis, there is no clinical role to palpating the carotid arteries; this is potentially hazardous and provides no useful diagnostic information.

Mental Status Testing of the Patient with Stroke

- When a disorder of language is suspected or when right-sided weakness is present, examine the patient for aphasia (see Chapter 6, Language Testing); the finding of aphasia is strong evidence of left hemispheric cortical involvement.
- In patients with left-sided weakness or in any patient with a suspicion for right hemisphere dysfunction, look for evidence of cortical involvement by testing for left-sided neglect. Neglect can be tested by asking the patient to draw a clock (see Chapter 8, Testing Orientation, Concentration, Knowledge, and Constructional Ability); patients with right parietal cortical dysfunction may neglect to fill in the numbers on the left side. You can also test for asomatognosia (neglect of the left side of the body) by holding the patient's left arm in front of his or her eyes and asking, "Whose arm is this?" Patients with asomatognosia may say the arm they see is the examiner's ("It's your arm") and not their own.

Cranial Nerve Examination of the Patient with Stroke

- Test visual fields to confrontation (see Chapter 13, Visual Field Examination). When a possible right hemispheric lesion is suspected, look for evidence of left-sided extinction on double simultaneous visual stimulation (see Chapter 31, Examination of Cortical Sensation), especially when a visual field deficit is not evident.

- Look for evidence of facial weakness (see Chapter 16, Examination of Facial Strength). Upper motor neuron facial weakness is seen in many patients with hemispheric strokes on the same side as the weak extremities. Lower motor neuron facial weakness can occur due to some pontine infarcts, often opposite to the side of extremity weakness as a crossed sign of brainstem dysfunction.

- Look at the optic fundi for the rare finding of Hollenhorst plaques (see Fig. 49–1); the finding of these cholesterol emboli supports the possibility of carotid disease, but the absence of this finding does not exclude it.

Motor Examination of the Patient with Stroke

- In patients without obvious severe weakness, look for drift of one of the outstretched arms as a subtle sign of weakness. When testing muscle strength in any patient with a possible stroke, concentrate on assessing for side-to-side asymmetries.

- Patients with weakness in the face and arm with relative preservation of leg strength most likely have infarction within the contralateral middle cerebral artery territory. Severe leg weakness due to stroke suggests involvement within the contralateral anterior cerebral artery territory.

- Patients with severe weakness involving the face, arm, and leg on one side of the body but no sensory or cortical symptoms or signs have a syndrome called *pure motor hemiparesis*. This finding is typical of a deep lesion, usually a lacunar infarct, affecting the motor fibers of the corticospinal tract, as they are concentrated together in the internal capsule or pons and segregated from other pathways; such extensive weakness would be difficult to attribute to a hemispheric cortical lesion without causing other nonmotor symptoms.

Sensory Examination of the Patient with Stroke

- Concentrate on assessing for significant side-to-side differences in sensation, such as to pin or gross touch.

- In patients with possible right hemisphere lesions, especially when no obvious sensory loss is seen, look for signs of right hemispheric cortical dysfunction by testing for left-sided extinction on double simultaneous stimulation, or other cortical sensory tests such as graphesthesia and stereognosis (see Chapter 31, Examination of Cortical Sensation).

- Patients with severe isolated hemisensory loss involving the face, arm, and leg on one side of the body are likely to have a thalamic stroke; these symptoms sometimes evolve to severe painful dysesthesias (called the *thalamic syndrome*).

Cerebellar Examination of the Patient with Stroke

- Dysmetria (see Chapter 33, Approach to the Cerebellar Examination) of the extremities on one side of the body, especially in the absence of weakness, suggests a cerebellar hemisphere stroke ipsilateral to the clumsy extremities. Some cerebellar strokes, however, particularly those involving the midline, may only have ataxia of gait with little if any dysmetria. Cerebellar strokes (infarction or hemorrhage) are important to recognize because they can become neurosurgical emergencies due to mass effect in the small space of the posterior fossa. Consider the possibility of cerebellar stroke in any patient with nausea, vomiting, or headache in the presence of difficulty with gait, regardless of whether there is dysmetria of the extremities.

- Prominent dysmetria of the extremities on one side of the body in the presence of mild weakness (or other corticospinal tract signs) on the same side is consistent with an ataxic-hemiparesis syndrome; this is usually due to a small infarct (usually a lacunar stroke) involving cerebellar pathway fibers and motor fibers within the contralateral internal capsule or pons (see Chapter 33, Approach to the Cerebellar Examination).

Reflex and Gait Examination of the Patient with Stroke

- Patients with hemispheric (deep or cortical) strokes or unilateral brainstem strokes can have a side-to-side reflex asymmetry, brisker on the weak side; however, such reflex changes might not be present acutely. A Babinski sign may be present on the weak side of any patient with a stroke causing motor weakness, even acutely.
- Patients with hemiparesis from a stroke usually have a characteristic hemiparetic gait, described in Chapter 39, Examination of Gait). Patients with cerebellar infarcts (or an ataxic-hemiparesis syndrome) often have an ataxic gait, falling to the side of the diseased cerebellar hemisphere, or may be unable to walk at all without falling.

ADDITIONAL COMMENTS

There are a few specific stroke syndromes not described above that deserve mentioning here:

- Patients with Wallenberg's syndrome have symptoms of vertigo, dysarthria, dysphagia, and unsteadiness. The examination shows diminished pin sensation on one side of the face and on the opposite side of the body, with findings of cerebellar ataxia, Horner's syndrome, and weakness of one side of the palate (see Fig. 19–1), all on the same side as the facial numbness. This classic, and not uncommon, syndrome results from an infarct of the lateral medulla.
- Gerstmann's syndrome consists of difficulty with writing (agraphia), calculations (acalculia), and finger naming (finger agnosia), with right/left confusion. This classic, but uncommon, stroke syndrome results from lesions involving the angular gyrus of the dominant posterior parietal lobe.

Chapter 53

EXAMINATION OF THE PATIENT WITHOUT NEUROLOGIC SYMPTOMS: THE SCREENING NEUROLOGIC EXAMINATION

PURPOSE OF THE SCREENING NEUROLOGIC EXAMINATION

The purpose of the examination of the patient without neurologic complaints is to look for evidence of unrecognized neurologic disease or the presence of unrecognized neurologic complications in a patient with a chronic systemic illness.

WHEN TO PERFORM THE SCREENING NEUROLOGIC EXAMINATION

A screening neurologic examination (in contrast to the thorough neurologic examination, as described in Chapter 40, Performing a Complete Neurologic Examination) should be performed as part of any comprehensive general medical examination.

NEUROANATOMY OF THE SCREENING NEUROLOGIC EXAMINATION

The basic relevant neuroanatomy underlying each examination element is briefly described in the chapters of Section 2, Neurologic Examination.

EQUIPMENT NEEDED TO PERFORM THE SCREENING NEUROLOGIC EXAMINATION

- An ophthalmoscope
- A reflex hammer
- 128-Hz tuning fork

HOW TO PERFORM THE SCREENING NEUROLOGIC EXAMINATION

Implementing the elements below, in the order shown, is one practical method of performing a screening neurologic examination in a typical patient without neurologic symptoms. If any abnormal findings are seen, then more detail should be included and more examination elements should be added, as indicated.

Mental Status

(In the patient without any neurologic complaints or symptoms and in whom there is no suspicion of a disorder of alertness, language, memory or any other aspect of cognition suggested during your history-taking, no formal evaluation of mental status is necessary.)

Examine the Cranial Nerves

1. Look at the resting size and symmetry of the pupils and examine the response of each pupil to light (see Chapter 10, Examination of the Pupils).

2. Perform a funduscopic examination to look at the optic discs (see Chapter 11, Funduscopic Examination); a funduscopic examination should be a routine part of any comprehensive medical examination.

3. Test visual fields to confrontation (see Chapter 13, Visual Field Examination). In the screening examination, this can be done quickly with both eyes open simultaneously and by just checking the left and the right visual fields (not the four quadrants).

4. Test horizontal eye movements and vertical eye movements (see Chapter 14, Examination of Eye Movements).

5. [Look for obvious facial asymmetry while you are talking to the patient, but unless obvious asymmetry is seen, there is probably no need to formally test facial strength (see Chapter 16, Examination of Facial Strength) in a screening examination.]

Examine Motor Function

6. Test for drift of the outstretched arms (see Chapter 25, Examination of Upper Extremity Muscle Strength).

7. Test the strength of a few upper extremity muscles (see Chapter 25, Examination of Upper Extremity Muscle Strength). In a simple screening examination of the patient with no neurologic complaints, it usually suffices to simply test one proximal and one distal muscle on each side, such as the deltoids (or biceps) and the interossei bilaterally.

8. Test the strength of a few lower extremity muscles (see Chapter 26, Examination of Lower Extremity Muscle Strength). In a simple screening examination, simply test one proximal and distal muscle on each side, such as the hip flexors (or the extensors at the knees) and the foot dorsiflexors bilaterally.

Examine Sensory Function

9. Test vibration sense in the toes (see Chapter 30, Examination of Vibration and Position Sensation).

Examine Cerebellar Function

10. Test the finger-to-nose maneuver (see Chapter 34, Testing of Upper Extremity Cerebellar Function).

Examine the Muscle Stretch Reflexes

11. Test the biceps jerks, triceps jerks, knee jerks, and ankle jerks (see Chapter 37, Examination of the Muscle Stretch Reflexes).

Examine for the Babinski Response

12. Test for the Babinski response on each foot (see Chapter 38, Testing for the Babinski Response).

Examine the Gait

13. If you haven't already informally observed the patient walking into the examination room, watch the patient walk a few steps (see Chapter 39, Examination of Gait).

NORMAL FINDINGS

Normal findings for each component of the neurologic examination are discussed in the chapters of Section 2, Neurologic Examination.

ABNORMAL FINDINGS

Abnormal findings for each component of the neurologic examination are discussed in the chapters of Section 2, Neurologic Examination. Any abnormalities found on a screening examination of a patient without neurologic symptoms should be interpreted with caution; it's usually best to err on the side of conservatism and try not to overinterpret subtle isolated findings.

Neurologic Tests

NEUROLOGIC IMAGING TESTS (COMPUTED TOMOGRAPHY AND MAGNETIC RESONANCE IMAGING)

Purpose

The main purpose of a neurologic imaging study is to look for evidence of a structural process involving the brain or spinal cord.

How the Test Works

Computed Tomography Scanning

Computed tomography (CT) is an x-ray–based study that differentiates structures based on their radiodensities. Lesions may show up as abnormal areas of hyperdensity (e.g., acute hemorrhage) or hypodensity (e.g., stroke, masses, or edema).

Magnetic Resonance Imaging Scanning

Magnetic resonance imaging (MRI) looks at how protons in tissues behave when subjected to a radiofrequency pulse after being aligned in a magnetic field. Several series of images are produced:

- T2 images are important because most pathologic processes appear bright (also called *high signal or hyperintense*) on these images.
- Most lesions are not as evident on T1 images, except for subacute blood.
- Fluid-attenuated inversion recovery (FLAIR) images are useful for visualizing lesions next to the ventricles.
- Diffusion-weighted images are sensitive for detecting early ischemic stroke.

Contrast-Enhanced Computed Tomography or Magnetic Resonance Imaging

Contrast agents enhance areas of blood–brain barrier breakdown and are useful when assessing tumors, abscesses, and acute ischemic or inflammatory lesions.

Computed Tomography Angiography and Magnetic Resonance Angiography

CT angiography and MR angiography provide noninvasive images of the extracranial and intracranial vessels.

When to Order Computed Tomography or Magnetic Resonance Imaging

Computed Tomography

- The main role for CT in neurologic diagnosis is in the emergency setting to look for evidence of an acute process involving the brain, especially for ruling out intracerebral hemorrhage in patients who present with an acute stroke syndrome or head trauma.
- CT is the first step in the evaluation of patients with possible acute subarachnoid hemorrhage (SAH), in which it is at least 90% sensitive.

Magnetic Resonance Imaging

- In the nonemergent setting and in the absence of contraindications, MRI is preferable to CT for most intracranial processes. Demyelination, small masses, and any lesion in the posterior fossa or sella especially are better seen on MRI.
- MRI is the most appropriate test in any patient who presents with symptoms or signs of spinal cord dysfunction because, unlike CT, MR images the cord well.
- Either MR angiography or CT angiography are options for noninvasive assessment of vascular stenosis in patients with possible cerebral ischemia or for noninvasive assessment of vascular malformations or for aneurysms larger than 3 mm in diameter.

NEUROPHYSIOLOGIC TESTS

Electromyography and Nerve Conduction Study

Purpose

The purpose of an electromyography (EMG)/nerve conduction study (NCS) is to look for electrophysiologic evidence of peripheral nervous system dysfunction.

How the Test Works

EMG and NCS are two separate components of the test and are performed in the same setting; the combination of both tests is often referred to simply as an *EMG*.

NERVE CONDUCTION STUDY

In the NCS, various motor and sensory nerves are stimulated with an electrical impulse to assess the velocity of conduction and the amplitude of the response.

- Slowing of conduction of a nerve is suggestive of peripheral nerve demyelination.
- Diminished motor or sensory amplitude suggests dysfunction of the nerve axon.
- A specialized NCS procedure, looking for a decrease in motor amplitude with repetitive nerve stimulation, can assist in the diagnosis of myasthenia gravis.

ELECTROMYOGRAPHY

In EMG, a needle electrode is inserted into various muscles, looking for evidence of abnormal electrical activity.

- The finding of fibrillations in a muscle suggests denervation to that muscle.
- Certain patterns of voluntary muscle contraction can help distinguish between neuropathic and myopathic processes.

When to Order an Electromyography and Nerve Conduction Study

EMG/NCS can be a helpful adjunct in the assessment of polyneuropathies, entrapment neuropathies, radiculopathies, myopathies, myasthenia gravis, and motor neuron disease.

Electroencephalography

Purpose

The main purpose of electroencephalography (EEG) is to look for electrophysiologic evidence of a seizure disorder.

How the Test Works

Electrodes are placed over the surface of the scalp to detect and record voltage differences between different areas of the brain.

- In many (but not all) patients with epilepsy, abnormal epileptiform patterns can be seen over the involved area of brain and can assist in determining whether the patient has a focal or primary generalized seizure disorder.
- EEG can also show a pattern called *triphasic waves* in some patients with metabolic (such as hepatic, uremic, or anoxic) encephalopathies.

When to Order an Electroencephalograph

- An EEG should be ordered in patients suspected of having epilepsy or in any comatose patient suspected of being in subclinical status epilepticus.
- An EEG may also be helpful in some encephalopathic patients, looking for triphasic waves as an additional clue to underlying metabolic dysfunction.

Lumbar Puncture and Cerebrospinal Fluid Analysis

Purpose

The main purpose of lumbar puncture (LP) and cerebrospinal fluid (CSF) analysis is to look for evidence of infectious, hemorrhagic (SAH), inflammatory/demyelinative, or neoplastic processes.

How the Test Works

An LP should not be performed in patients who have a space-occupying lesion in the brain due to the risk of herniation; typically, this should be excluded by brain imaging. To perform an LP, the L-4 to L-5 interspace is sterilely entered with a spinal needle. An opening pressure should be obtained, and CSF studies should typically include cell count, protein, glucose, Gram stain, and cultures. Depending on the indication, other studies can include cytology, immunoglobulin G/albumin ratio, oligoclonal bands, VDRL, cryptococcal antigen, and specific polymerase chain reaction tests and cultures.

- An elevated opening pressure (>200 mm H_2O) is consistent with increased intracranial pressure.
- Elevated number of white blood cells (typically >5/mm³) is consistent with an infectious (e.g., meningitis) or inflammatory process.
- Increased number of red blood cells, especially with xanthochromia (yellowish tinge to the supernatant after CSF is spun down), would be consistent with SAH.
- Diminished glucose (<60% of simultaneous blood glucose) can be seen in bacterial as well as some other meningitides.
- Elevated CSF protein (>45 mg/dL) is nonspecific and can be seen in a variety of processes. A classic finding in demyelinating polyneuropathies, such as the Guillain-Barré syndrome, is an elevated protein without pleocytosis, however.
- Elevated immunoglobulin G/albumin ratio (e.g., >0.30) or the presence of oligoclonal bands may be seen with inflammatory or demyelinating processes, such as multiple sclerosis.

When to Perform a Lumbar Puncture and Cerebrospinal Fluid Analysis

- LP should be performed in patients suspected of having meningitis and in patients who are suspected of having an SAH despite a negative CT.

- LP can also be helpful in the assessment of patients with possible inflammatory or demyelinative processes in the central or peripheral nervous system.
- An LP with opening pressure should also be obtained in patients suspected of having pseudotumor cerebri.

INDEX

Page numbers followed by *f* indicate figures; numbers followed by *t* indicate tables.